*Psychiatric*
*Polarities*

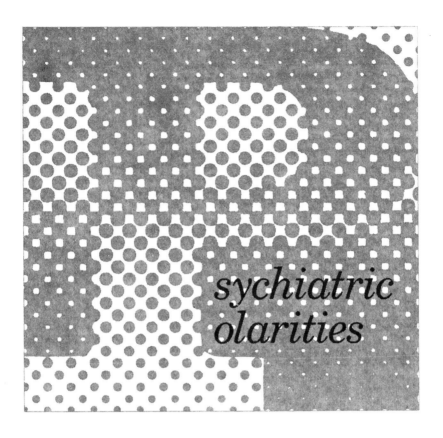
*sychiatric olarities*

# Methodology & Practice

Phillip R. Slavney, M.D.
& Paul R. McHugh, M.D.

Johns Hopkins University Press
Baltimore

For our parents

This book was published with the generous assistance of
the Department of Psychiatry and Behavioral Sciences,
Johns Hopkins University School of Medicine.

Johns Hopkins University Press
2715 North Charles Street
Baltimore, Maryland 21218-4363
www.press.jhu.edu

*The Library of Congress has cataloged the hardcover edition
of this book as follows:*

Slavney, Phillip R. (Phillip Richard), 1940–
    Psychiatric polarities.
    Bibliography: p.
    Includes index.
    1. Psychiatry—Philosophy. 2. Polarity. I. McHugh,
Paul R. (Paul Rodney), 1931– . II. Title. [DNLM: 1. Mental
Disorders. 2. Philosophy, Medical. 3. Psychiatry—methods.
WM 100 S6313p]

RC 437.5.S55     1987          616.89'001      86-21446
ISBN 0-8018-3428-7 (hardcover : alk. paper)

ISBN 978-1-4214-1976-3 (pbk : alk. paper)
ISBN 978-1-4214-1977-0 (electronic)

*Special discounts are available for bulk purchases of this
book. For more information, please contact Special Sales at
410-516-6936 or specialsales@press.jhu.edu.*

# Contents

# Preface

It is a tendency of human beings to think in terms of polar opposites: day and night, hot and cold, appearance and reality, thought and action, cause and effect, Apollonian and Dionysian—the list could go on and on. Thinking in this way has several attractive features. For one thing, it makes complicated issues appear simple. Orators have long known that reducing an ambiguous and controversial subject to a pair of antithetical ideas is an effective rhetorical technique. Then too, the juxtaposition of opposites creates a tension that is stimulating. In music, we find the alternation of loud and soft; in painting, the contrast between light and shade; in literature, the struggle of good with evil. Indeed, when the clash of opposites is presented as it is in professional wrestling—good and evil shorn of all ambiguity—the emotional arousal produced can be quite powerful, as anyone who has ever observed the crowd (or him-or herself) at such a spectacle will confirm.

In psychiatry, the polarizations are less violent than they are in wrestling, but they arouse our passions just the same. Mind and brain, conscious and unconscious, patient and client: such polarities define fields of conflict as much as they do spheres of interest. Why should this be so? And why should some disagreements in psychiatry take the form of philosophical disputes rather than scientific debates?

We hope this examination of several important psychiatric polarities will help to answer such questions. Most of the essays composing this book begin with a clinical issue that illustrates the polarity at hand. The polarity's place in the history of ideas is then considered, and following that, the polarity is discussed in the light of psychiatric methodology and practice. Because the issues discussed are controversial ones, we have presented a number of direct quotations from primary sources. Our purpose in this was not only to let authors speak for themselves, lest we distort their views, but also to acquaint readers with observations and proposals as they were originally made.

This book is intended to illustrate our opinion that psychiatry is a bridging discipline between the biological sciences and the humanities and that it takes from both in the excitement of its controversies. Our viewpoint is derived from the clinic, however, rather than from the laboratory or the classroom, and the controversies arise as we care for patients rather than as we design experiments or defend theses. This clinical perspective is thrust upon us by the reality of illness, and it will not disappear, despite advances in the sciences and the humanities, because patients will remain both organisms *and* agents, both objects *and* subjects. It is for this reason that psychiatry has much to learn from the sciences and from the humanities, but it is also for this reason that psychiatry has much to teach.

We are indebted to Marshal Folstein, Mark Komrad, Neil Pauker, Anders Richter, and Jacqueline Slavney for their critical readings of our manuscript and for their valuable counsel.

Some support for this work was provided by the National Institute of Mental Health Comprehensive Institutional Training Grant MH17288.

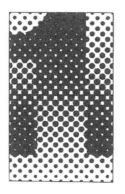

*The
Ambiguity of
Psychiatry*

# 1

# Psychiatry's Domain

In *The Perspectives of Psychiatry* we discussed the methods of clinical reasoning basic to the field.[1] Our aim was to help students think critically about the opinions offered within psychiatry, and thereby enable them to transcend the denominational conflicts that impede it. In this book we will examine some of those conflicts more closely and try again to demonstrate how a methodological approach—one that considers the procedures by which ideas are generated—can help resolve disagreements rooted in partisan commitments.

Thinking methodologically is important because psychiatry is an ambiguous discipline. Though its ambiguity can be appreciated at many levels, it is perhaps most evident to beginners when they try to define psychiatry's domain of interest, when they try to answer the question: "Where exactly do psychiatrists look for the signs and symptoms on which they base their diagnoses and treatments?"

This is an intriguing question, in part because psychiatrists are the only physicians of whom it is asked. Would anyone wonder about the domain of interest of an ophthalmologist or a dermatologist, for example? The eye and the skin are so immediately objects of study in their own right that the question never arises. What psychiatrists look at and where it is are more puzzling issues.

Psychiatrists themselves seem to have difficulty defining their province. Some are interested in mental states, others in behavior, and still others in the person. On reflection, though, most psychiatrists would agree that they look for signs and symptoms in the domain of personal consciousness, in a realm we might call the "phenomenal world."

## The Phenomenal World

The phenomenal world is the most immediate and vivid experience of human beings. It contains not only our perceptions, emotions, and intentions but also that sense of self, of "me-ness" that gives our existence identity and continuity. These characteristics of the phenomenal world can all be identified in the following passage by the Gestalt psychologist Wolfgang Köhler, who describes a realm of personal consciousness that

> consists, at this moment, of a blue lake with dark forests around it, a big, gray stone, hard and cool, which I have chosen as a chair, a paper on which I write, a faint noise of the wind which hardly moves the trees, and a strong odor characteristic of boats and fishing. But there is more in this world: somehow I now behold, though it does not become fused with the blue lake of the present, another lake of a milder blue, and I find myself, some years ago, looking at it from its shore in Illinois. I am perfectly accustomed to beholding thousands of pictures of this kind which arise some way or other when I am alone. And there is still more in this world: my hand and fingers moving lightly over the smooth surface of the paper; now, when I stop writing and look around again, there is a feeling of health and vigor, but in the next moment I feel something like a dark pressure somewhere in my interior which tends to develop into a feeling of being hunted—I have promised to have this manuscript ready within a few months. [2]

Although the phenomenal world Köhler describes is a private one, in that only he can experience it, the nature of his experience can be made public through the language we share with him. The phenomenal world, unique for each of us but common to us all, is psychiatry's domain.

And yet, to say this is immediately to raise important issues. Work in the phenomenal world must face several challenges, such as the fallibility of introspection, the cultural barriers to communication, and the effect of theory on what is considered trivial and what significant. Even if these difficulties are acknowledged, however, the domain itself is suspect. It is not like the eye or the skin. It has no "place." And though it may be granted that the phenomenal world is "located" within the patient, we must admit that it is not a *world* at all, not a *thing*, but rather a metaphor for our experience.

Still, that experience is real, and whether we call it the "phenomenal world" or something else, it is the point of contact between psychiatrists and their patients. Indeed, the phenomenal world is much more than that: it is the starting point for all knowledge, whether of ourselves or of the universe around us.[3]

Psychiatrists not only look for signs and symptoms in the phenomenal world but turn to it again and again in order to judge the reliability of their diagnoses and the efficacy of their treatments. Though behavioral observations and laboratory tests can help in these matters, they cannnot replace the psychiatric history and mental status examination, in which we "map" the patient's phenomenal world, past and present, by discriminating among the experiences it contains and deciding which are significant for the issue at hand.

But as physicians, we want to do more than depict the phenomenal world: we want to account for its disturbances and understand its foundations. To explain the patient's complaints, we must sometimes look beyond the phenomenal world itself. The first thing to strike us as we do so is that mental life is dependent on the brain: thoughts and moods do not occur without neurons and synapses. Yet mind and brain are not identical. Indeed, they are so different that the nature of their relationship is the fundamental mystery in psychiatry and the source of many of its conflicts.

**The Essential Polarity**

At the frontier of brain and mind, the referents we use change from tangibles, such as neurons and synapses, to intangibles, such as thoughts and moods. The boundary thus represents a point of disjunction rather than fusion; in crossing it, we suddenly move from the realm of matter to the realm of experience, from the world of bodies to the world of selves. Though we know that mental life and brain processes are related, we do not know how to account for one in terms of the other. Synthetic explanations from the neuron up and reductionistic analyses from the thought down do not meet. Instead, they leave a gap so wide that the most meaningful characteristic of the phenomenal world—its subjective sense of self— remains disconnected from the objectively demonstrated dependence of that self on the central nervous system.

Because of the disjunction between mind and brain, the phenomenal world *must* be viewed from several different perspectives if it is to be fully appreciated. It can, for example, be disrupted both by the onset of a process in the patient's brain and by the meaning of an event in his life. We eventually explain the first type of disturbance through knowledge of the material world; we immediately understand the second through fellow-feeling. There is no way in which such differing approaches can be fully integrated, no "unified field theory" that contains all the concepts and information needed in psychiatric practice. Though psychoanalysis, behaviorism, and the neurosciences have all claimed to provide such a framework, none has succeeded in doing so.

These concepts fail to unite mind and brain not because they are insufficiently developed but because they cannot make the transition from the machinery of the brain to the experience of the mind. They cannot cross the gap except in metaphorical terms, or, like Watsonian behaviorism, they must repudiate its existence by denying the reality of mental life itself.

Mind and brain can neither be fully integrated nor completely separated. This fact, more than anything else, accounts for psychiatry's ambiguity and controversy. Mind and brain are not only different viewpoints on the phenomenal world and its disturbances, they are thesis and antithesis, polar opposites in a dialectic about the essential nature of human beings.

## Some Consequences of the Polarity of Mind and Brain

Because the polarity of mind and brain is so fundamental a problem in psychiatric methodology, its consequences are found throughout the field. If, for example, the experiences of the phenomenal world could be reduced to brain processes, the methods of the natural sciences would be adequate to explain all psychiatric disorders. Since mental life is more than the sum of brain events, however, since human beings exist in a world of meaning as well as in a world of matter, the methods of the humanities are indispensable if certain phenomena are to be appreciated. The tension between the methods of the natural sciences and the methods of the humanitites thus forms another polarity in psychiatric thought, which will be explored in the chapter on *explanation* and *understanding*.

But even if the humanities bring a greater appreciation of the phenomenal world than is possible from the viewpoint of science alone, much remains that is baffling. Why, for example, should a patient choose to behave in a certain way when it seems so self-defeating? Why should he repeatedly establish relationships that end in disappointment, or continue to drink alcohol at the risk of death? The patient is disturbed and puzzled by his behavior yet is unable to stop it. Neither the patient's conscious deliberation nor the psychiatrist's empathic understanding seems to expose the roots of the problem. In such circumstances, the existence of unconscious conflicts may be proposed, and with them comes all the controversy surrounding the polarity of conscious and unconscious factors in mental life.

The phenomenal world is the domain of the self. Though we know that brain mechanisms and unconscious processes determine to some extent the potentials and decisions of human beings, our conscious experience is that, in the end, to a greater or lesser degree, our behavior is "self"-directed—that we are free to choose, and that we can be held responsible for our choices. This experience of the deciding self in the phenomenal world may be an illusion, but it is an illusion by which we all live.

In the course of discovering why their choices have been so troublesome, patients often ask their psychiatrists, "Have you ever dealt with this problem before?" and "Am I the only one who acts this way?" The answers given to such questions reveal another facet of the mind—brain polarity: human beings are both singular and similar. Though their phenomenal worlds and life histories are unique, their potentials for experience and behavior are shaped into certain patterns by the resemblance of their brains and by the templates of their cultures. The contrast between seeing the patient as an individual and seeing him as a representative human type is discussed in the polarity of *Hebraic* and *Hellenic*.

How psychiatrists regard their patients is not only a question of knowledge but of values, not only a matter of facts but of meanings. The psychiatrist-patient relationship is perhaps more controversial than other medical relationships because of psychiatry's inherent ambiguity. If all of us were only psychotherapists (and dealt with the mind) or simply neuroscientists (and dealt with the brain), there might be less discord about our practice. As it is, psychiatrists must comprehend and treat patients whose minds are distressed and those whose brains are diseased, patients whose choices are damaging and those whose capacity to choose has been damaged, patients who desire our help and ask for it, and those who desperately need our assistance but repudiate it. What constitutes a proper professional relationship is thus a vexing issue, and we will examine two aspects of it under the polarities of patient-client and autonomy-paternalism.

## Conclusion

Despite the ambiguity and complexity of psychiatry, it is striking that many students begin its study with the appearance of having already solved its greatest mysteries. They declare themselves champions of the mind or defenders of the brain and are prepared from the first to argue about almost anything. They want to learn how to care for patients but not to have their assumptions challenged.

Perhaps this should not be surprising, given that psychiatry is a discipline in which one's professional identity can be defined as much by what he repudiates as by what he affirms. Psychiatrists, after all, are the only physicians regularly said to have this or that "orientation," and the labels affixed mark them as friend or foe. In order not to be wounded before they even know what the fight is about, beginning students may seek protection in one or another warring camp. The unfortunate result is that many of them become partisans—and needless casualties—in denominational conflicts that have gone on for generations and that they scarcely understand.

In our exploration of the mind-brain polarity and some of its consequences, we will try to demonstrate how a methodological approach can illuminate the foundations of dogma. We are not opposed to certainty or to advocacy as such (for many things *are* established and, as you will see, we have opinions of our own) but rather to the unreflective acceptance of doctrinaire positions as a means of resolving ambiguity. Psychiatry needs more light and less heat, or it will remain a battleground "where ignorant armies clash by night." We hope this book will be illuminating.

# 2
# Mind
# & Brain

## Grief

It usually begins with words: "Carol, I have some terrible news. Charles was in an accident—a very bad accident. I'm afraid he's been killed."

Those words, that information imparted in a few seconds, change the hearer's life. At first she is stunned and unable to accept the fact: "There must be some mistake. Charles is a good driver. He's never had an accident. He's just badly hurt. He can't be dead."

This state of numbness and disbelief characterizes the first hours or days of bereavement, but it eventually gives way to a feeling of anxious distress and to pangs of grief, episodes in which "the lost person is strongly missed and the survivor sobs or cries aloud for him."[1] During these spells of pining, of intense yearning for the deceased, the survivor's phenomenal world is filled with thoughts of the lost person and the circumstances of his death. The bereaved individual is usually restless, may search the environment for signs of the deceased, and is alerted by sounds that could herald his return. As well, the survivor experiences insomnia, poor appetite, distractibility, loss of interest in daily activities, and apparently unwarranted outbursts of anger at family and friends.

After several weeks or months of sad and irritable yearning, the bereaved individual is increasingly able to accept the fact of her loss and to begin the process of redefining her life. At times she is overcome by despair and apathy, but if all goes well the survivor starts to act as a widow rather than a wife; as a single person rather than a spouse. More is involved in this process than the experience

and expression of emotion. In John Bowlby's opinion, the "redefinition of self and situation is no mere release of affect but a cognitive
act on which all else turns."[2]

This is the uncomplicated acute grief reaction. Though it is
more complex than we have sketched, and though the mourning
behavior that accompanies it is culturally influenced, the essence
of the grief reaction is recognizable across the ages in the historical,
literary, and medical writings of many peoples. As Bowlby notes:
"Social custom differs enormously. Human response stays much the
same" (p.126).

How are we best to comprehend normal grief? On the one hand,
it cannot occur without a relationship, without emotional attachment, without love. Loss without love may produce regret but never
grief. Further, grief starts with information, with a message. The
pattern of sound waves that carries the grief-bringing message may
differ little from that which brings solace ("He is dead." "He isn't
dead."), but in that difference lies a world of human significance.
It is the meaning of the information that is important, and its meaning to someone in particular. Thus, though two people hear the same
words, one is grief-stricken and the other is untouched. Looked at
in this way, grief is best understood in terms of love, loss, meaning,
and the redefinition of a life; in terms of emotions, reactions, and
intentions; in terms of mental functions and experiences.

On the other hand, the potential for grief is universal among
human beings, which suggests that it is linked in some important
way to our biological makeup. This view is supported by consid-
erable evidence for the occurrence of grief or grieflike reactions in
nonhuman species.[3] Further, the changes in mood, thinking, behavior, and bodily functions that characterize grief are similar to
those found in affective disorders,[4] and it has even been proposed
that, because of its regular manifestations and predictable course,
grief might properly be regarded as a syndrome, or even as a disease.[5] Indeed, there is ample proof that bereavement is associated
with poor health,[6] increased mortality,[7] and even with a specific
mechanism (supression of the immune system) that could account
for illness and death among survivors.[8]

Perhaps Bowlby's "redefinition of self and situation" is only the
appearance of choice, an illusion in the phenomenal world, the out-
ward expression of brain processes that preceed and determine all
thought. Looked at in this way, grief might be better explained as
a biologically based disorder, as a succession of states in the brain

which transmutes all experience, as a matter of neurophysiology and neurochemistry.

The issue of grief and how we are to view it confronts the polarity of mind and brain, and we now return to that intriguing subject.

## The Polarity of Mind and Brain

In the late nineteenth century there was great hope that psychiatric disorders would be explained through study of the brain and its diseases. After all, Pierre Paul Broca and Karl Wernicke had demonstrated that damage to particular regions of the brain could produce specific psychological deficits (aphasias), and the discovery that general paresis was the result of a syphilitic infestation of the brain had revealed a discrete cause for a devastating mental disorder. Though there were cautionary voices at the time—Franz Nissl, for example, warned against a "brain mythology"[9] — psychiatric disorders were seen by many physicians as diseases of the brain and thus as amenable to the methods of the natural sciences.

By the early years of this century, however, it was evident that a brain-based approach had failed to account for many psychiatric conditions, and some physicians began to look more closely at the phenomenal world itself for clues to the genesis and treatment of mental disturbances. The person most closely identified with this shift in emphasis is Sigmund Freud, whose own attempts to explain mental events by cerebral processes had been unsuccessful (as in the *Project for a Scientific Psychology* of 1895). Freud then began to concentrate more on the meaning of mental experiences than on their relationship to neurological function; he began to use empathy rather than experiment as a way of understanding psychiatric disorders.

To Adolf Meyer, the tendency to think about psychiatry in terms of "brain" *or* "mind" was most unfortunate. He believed that the "object of our study is, literally, an *indivisible individual*. To be more explicit, it is a unit of biology which functions always as a 'he' or 'she' or person, by itself and in groups."[10] This view was the basis for Meyer's concept, "psychobiology," in which persons are seen as beings integrated in their physiological and psychological functioning:

We need no longer make a fatal chasm in the world of our experience, an irrevocable contrast between materialism and spirituality. We find it easier and truer to fact to view the "he" or "she," the "you" or "I" as the product of a natural development, with physics and chemistry blossoming through a biological organization into the human time-bound and time-consuming natural history entity, the person, who not only breathes in the service of the oxygen-carbon dioxide exchange, but also uses his breath in the unit functions of speech and song. . . . The symbolizing or meaning functions of the human being are as necessary to the maintenance of its life as are its physiological part-functions, and in a science of nature including man we have to find a place for them. In psychobiology we meet this challenge by specifying a domain with its own distinctive relations and calling for its own definite working methods and concepts. (P. 64)

Thus, for Meyer, "the person" was a level of biological organization just as important for clinical reasoning as other levels, such as the molecular or the cellular. Functioning at each level has its own rules and should be studied in its own terms.

Despite Meyer's views, however, "mind" and "brain" have generally been regarded as competing rather than complementary perspectives on the phenomenal world and its disturbances. Indeed, little seems to have changed since 1912, when E. E. Southard observed:

Some years ago I ventured from my chosen path of brain analysis in mental disease at large to a discussion of dementia precox in particular. I found that practically everybody had taken sides. It had become a game: the hypothesis of psychic factors was strictly opposed to the hypothesis of encephalic factors. Tangles and twists in the mind appealed to some: blots and spots in the brain appealed to others.[11]

Throughout the twentieth century, supporters of the "mind twist" and "brain spot" approaches have struggled for dominance in psychiatry. At certain times, and in certain places, one or the other has emerged victorious and has carried with it a generation of followers. In the United States of the 1950s, for example, most of the influential psychiatrists were psychoanalysts, as a matter of course; in the United States of the 1980s, their successors are likely to be neuroscientists. Because the sense of allegiance is so strong and the stakes in power and prestige so high, the polarization between these viewpoints has often been complete. It is no wonder that beginners in psychiatry have felt compelled to join one or another camp, to become either "mind doctors" or "brain doctors."

This schism in psychiatry is but the reflection of a larger polarity of mind and brain, one that calls into question the nature of human existence. Should people be thought of as subjects or objects? Agents or organisms? Selves or machines? Although these questions have engaged profound and imaginative thinkers for centuries, they are as fresh today as they ever were.

In the following sections we examine several major viewpoints on the polarity of mind and brain. Our goal is not to review the entire philosophical debate but to illustrate some of the opinions that inform the issue for psychiatry and its practice. We do not consider theories, such as methodological behaviorism, that deny the reality of mental experience, nor do we examine those, like idealism, that deny the reality of matter. It is clear to us that the phenomenal world is real and that it is dependent upon the brain for its existence.

PSYCHONEURAL IDENTITY THEORY

The first approach to the polarity of mind and brain we will summarize is the psychoneural identity theory, a point of view that has its roots in a materialist concept of the universe dating from ancient Greece. Philosophers and scientists have successfully used materialism to explain the world around them, so it is understandable that they would turn to it as they seek to explain the world within them.

The central tenet of the psychoneural identity theory is that mental experiences are brain processes, and nothing more. In the words of J. J. C. Smart:

When I say that a sensation is a brain process or that lightning is an electric discharge, I am using "is" in the sense of strict identity. (Just as in the—in this case necessary—proposition "7 is identical with the smallest prime number greater than 5.") When I say that a sensation is a brain process or that lightning is an electric discharge I do not mean just that the sensation is somehow spatially or temporally continuous with the brain process or that the lightning is just spatially or temporally continuous with the discharge. . . . I wish to make it clear that the brain-process doctrine asserts identity in the *strict* sense.[12]

The fundamental assumption behind the psychoneural identity theory is that there is nothing in the universe

but increasingly complex arrangements of physical constituents. All except for one place: in consciousness. That is, for a full description of what is going on in a man you would have to mention not only the physical processes in his tissues . . . but also his states of consciousness. . . . That these should be *correlated* with brain processes does not help, for to say that they are *correlated* is to say that they are something "over and above." . . . So sensations, states of consciousness, do seem to be the one sort of thing left outside the physicalist picture, and for various reasons I just cannot believe that this can be so. That everything should be explicable in terms of physics . . . except the occurrence of sensations seems to me to be frankly unbelievable. (P. 161)

Thus, according to the identity theory, there is only matter and energy. Mental experience is not denied but is considered isomorphic with brain processes. There is no separate, immaterial realm of psychological forces that somehow (perhaps through violating the principle of the conservation of energy) effect changes in the physical realm. Mind-brain interaction is, rather, brain-brain interaction.

This proposal is a seductive one, for it promises that the phenomenal world will be explained as nothing more than neuronal activity, a topic we already know something about. It is only a matter of time, so the argument goes, only a matter of modeling neural systems more complex than those we now comprehend.

And yet the events of the phenomenal world *as such* do not emerge from a greater knowledge of the material world—not even a material world composed of neurons, synapses, and neurotransmitters dynamically interrelated. What must be explained is how the phenomenal world *as experienced by the subject* can be derived from neural events. The identity theory does not tell us that, nor does any materialist viewpoint on the polarity of mind and brain, including emergentist materialism, which tries to avoid the identity theory's reductionist approach.

EMERGENTIST MATERIALISM

The general concept of "emergence" became popular in the early decades of this century as an alternative to mechanistic and reductionistic views of evolution. Thus C. Lloyd Morgan, one of its first champions, wrote in 1926:

We live in a world in which there seems to be an orderly sequence of events. It is the business of science . . . to describe the course of events . . . and to discover the plan on which they proceed. Evolution, in the broad sense of the word, is the name we give to the comprehensive plan of sequence in all natural events.

But the orderly sequence, historically viewed, appears to present, from time to time, something genuinely new. Under what I here call emergent evolution stress is laid on this incoming of the new. Salient examples are afforded in the advent of life, in the advent of mind, and in the advent of reflective thought. . . .

The naturalistic contention is that, on the evidence, not only atoms and molecules, but organisms and minds are susceptible of treatment by scientific methods fundamentally of like kind; that all belong to one tissue of events; and that all exemplify one foundational plan. In other words the position is that, in a philosophy based on the procedure sanctioned by progress in scientific research and thought, the advent of novelty of any kind is loyally to be accepted wherever it is found, without invoking any extra-natural Power (Force, Entelechy, Elan, or God) through the efficient Activity of which the observed facts may be explained.[13]

Opinions such as these engaged leading psychologists of the day, some of whom criticized the emergentist position as an attempt to find a way between the Scylla of mechanistic materialism and the Charybdis of teleology. And yet the theory continued to attract adherents, not only among those who wished to account for the appearance of mental life in animals but also among those who believed that integration might be as scientific a principle as reduction, especially in biology.

A contemporary statement of emergentist materialism is found in the writings of Mario Bunge:

Emergentist materialism . . . holds that the CNS [central nervous system], far from being a physical entity—in particular a machine—is a biosystem, i.e. a complex thing endowed with properties and laws peculiar to living things and, moreover, *very* peculiar ones, i.e. not shared by all bio-systems. . . .

The emergence claimed for the mental is double: the mental properties of a CNS are not possessed by its cellular components but are *systemic properties* and, moreover, nonresultant ones; and they have emerged *at some point in time* in the course of a long biotic evolutionary process. . . . Consequently, although physics and chemistry are necessary to explain CNS functions, they are insufficient. Nor does general biology suffice: we need to know the *specific emergent* properties and laws of the CNS, not only those it shares with other subsystems of the animal, such as the cardiovascular and the digestive systems. . . .

Reductive materialism [the psychoneural identity theory] . . . holds that the brain is nothing but an aggregate of cells, so that knowing the latter is not only necessary but also sufficient for knowing the former and thus explaining the mental. This reductionistic thesis is false. . . . A brain is a system, hence something endowed with a structure and an environment, not only a composition. And the structure of the brain includes the connections among its neurons. The result is a system with emergent properties—such as those of being able to perceive, feel, re-member, imagine, will, think, and others—which its cellular components lack.[14]

This is a vigorous denial of reductionistic materialism—what Roger Sperry called "an infinite nihilistic regress in which even-tually everything is held to be explainable in terms of essentially nothing"[15]—but it is materialism nonetheless. Bunge explains men-tal experiences such as willing and mental states like self-aware-ness as the activities of "plastic" neural systems (i.e., those whose functions have not been genetically determined). He asserts the identity of mental events and brain events and denies existence to "the mind" as a noncorporeal entity. For Bunge, as for other ma-terialists, mind-brain interactions cannot occur because mutual ef-fects are possible only between concrete things.

In Bunge's view, dualism (the proposition that mind and brain are two entities on the same footing) has impeded the resolution of the mind-brain problem because it has posited something (a myth grounded in an ideology) that is not amenable to the scientific method. He admits that emergentist materialism has not resolved the problem either, but he is optimistic that it will do so because it encourages scientists to behave as scientists, "not as amateur phi-losophers or theologians."[16]

The question is, What is it to behave as a scientist? Part of scientific behavior is to look behind the appearances of things. In that way, our everyday knowledge of the world, which is based on appearances (e.g., the sun rises in the East), is eventually brought into line with another state of knowledge. So, it is claimed by ma-terialists, our mentalistic concepts and language (e.g., "I made up my mind." "I was of two minds about it.") will become, like the flat earth idea, of interest only to historians.

Yet part of scientific behavior is also to keep an open mind about the nature of things, to make assumptions and to test them by ex-ploring their consequences. This is the process of conjectural ex-planation in science, and it is to be contrasted to that of essentialist explanation.[17] In the latter method, the nature of things is defined in advance, and from that premise all phenomena of interest are deduced. If some things cannot be accounted for in this way, the premise itself is rarely questioned, but rather the inventiveness, skill, or energy of the scientist.

A materialist who reasons from the essentialist method takes as his premise the idea that the universe contains nothing but matter and energy. What cannot be deduced from that premise is considered either a problem too complex to be solved by current materialist theory and technology (e.g., which brain systems interact to account for the mental state of grief) or not a problem for science at all, since the phenomena in question (e.g., "mental" states) cannot exist.

This approach to the mind-brain issue can be very persuasive to beginners in psychiatry. For one thing, it seems so natural. Materialism does not demand a radical shift in thinking but builds on the assumptions of many science courses that students have already taken at university and medical school. Further, as noted above, growing knowledge about the brain seems to promise a resolution of psychiatry's ambiguity, if not just now, then at least in the foreseeable future. It is perhaps this sense of continuity with a powerful and successful tradition in science that accounts for the confidence of many materialists as they argue their case, and for the fact that so many students of psychiatry defend materialism's claims without having thought very deeply about its axioms or its consequences.

If we can step back from the premises of materialism in our examination of the mind-brain polarity, however, and if we can remember that all knowledge, scientific or otherwise, begins with the phenomenal world, we may find ourselves pondering not only the structure and function of the nervous system but also questions like "What is the nature of experience?" and "How might an interaction between mind and brain be characterized, assuming they were separate entities?"

The answer to the first question seems clear: the nature of experience (the phenomenal world) is dualistic. We are aware of both our minds and our bodies, and we are often much more aware of the former than the latter. We experience deciding, willing, concentrating, and anticipating not in our bodies or brains but somewhere in the phenomenal world (though we often experience our "selves," as when writing or reading, just behind our eyes). Indeed, we can imagine ourselves to be ourselves even if we were embodied in a cat, in a stone, or in nothing at all. And even the most materialistic scientist, even the most radical behaviorist, experiences the world as if his mind controlled his body, not the other way around. Existential duality is a fact, and if we are to avoid the trap of the essentialist method, we must conjecture about the nature of that fact.

The second problem—how to characterize an interaction between mind and brain—does not acknowledge the claims of several dualist viewpoints (e.g., that mind and brain are parallel but independent of one another). We have chosen psychoneural interactionism to illustrate mind-brain dualism in part because it brings the issues into sharpest focus and in part because it occasioned one of the most celebrated conjectures in the history of science and philosophy.

PSYCHONEURAL INTERACTIONISM

René Descartes postulated an incorporeal soul and a mechanical body, but he needed a point of contact between them:

As a beginning, I will answer the question you asked me about the function of the little gland called *conarion* [the pineal]. My view is that this gland is the principal seat of the soul, and the place in which all our thoughts are formed. The reason I believe this is that I cannot find any part of the brain, except this, which is not double. Since we see only one thing with two eyes, and hear only one voice with two ears, and altogether have only one thought at a time, it must necessarily be the case that the impressions which enter by the two eyes or by the two ears, and so on, unite with each other in some part of the body before being considered by the soul. Now it is impossible to find any such place, in the whole head, except this gland; moreover it is situated in the most suitable possible place for this purpose, in the middle of all the concavities; and it is supported and surrounded by the little branches of the carotid arteries which bring the spirits into the brain.[18]

Though Descartes believed in ultimate explanations about the nature of human beings, he also knew about neuroanatomy and tried to defend his views on the localization of the mind-brain interaction by appealing to empirical evidence:

The difficulty you raise about the *conarium* seems to be most urgent. . . . So without waiting for the next post I will say that the pituitary gland is akin to the pineal gland in that both are situated between the carotid arteries and on the path which the spirits take in rising from the heart to the brain. But this gives no ground to suppose that the two have the same function; for the pituitary gland is not, like the pineal gland, in the brain, but beneath it and entirely separate, in a concavity of the sphenoid bone specially made to take it, and even beneath the *dura mater* if I remember correctly. Moreover, it is entirely immobile, whereas we experience, when we imagine, that the seat of the common sense, that is to say the part of the brain in which the soul performs all its principal operations, must be mobile. (P. 85)

The seat of the soul had to be mobile so that it could impart motion to the "animal spirits," which in turn would transmit that motion to the nerves and muscles of the body. For the body to communicate with the soul, the process was reversed. The pineal gland, which is mobile to a small degree, seemed well-suited to the purpose.

Where does the contact between mind and brain occur? By what means does the reciprocal influence take place? These questions are central to any interactionist theory. Though Descartes was wrong about the pineal, he faced the questions squarely.

A much-discussed interactionist proposal has recently been made by Karl Popper and John Eccles.[19] We will not review here Popper's philosophical contribution to their theory but will focus instead on the neurophysiological argument of Eccles, which is in the Cartesian tradition.

At the core of mental life in human beings is the unity of conscious experience, the "self or the ego that is the basis of the personal identity and continuity that each of us experiences throughout our lifetime" (p. 360). Eccles believes that this unity of experience cannot be accounted for by the brain's neural machinery alone. Brain events are discontinuous and disparate; they need something to integrate them. This integrative function is carried out by the mind, which is developed to give unity to the conscious self.

Eccles proposed a point of contact between mind and brain which was suggested by the work of Sperry and his associates with commissurotomy patients:

From this evidence there is derived the concept that only a specialized zone of the cerebral hemispheres is in liaison with the self-conscious mind. The term liaison brain denotes all those areas of the cerebral cortex that potentially are capable of being in direct liasion with the self-conscious mind. . . . In the commissurotomy patient this liaison brain is restricted to the dominant hemisphere, presumably encompassing the linguistic areas of that hemisphere, though doubtless extending more widely to encompass areas that are concerned with non-verbal modes of conscious experiences. . . . However, normally there may well be some liaison areas of brain in the minor hemisphere. (P. 358)

The mind exerts its integrating function by "reading out" neural activities in the liaison brain, by "scanning" and "probing" modules of cortical neurons. The mind selects from these modules based on current interests, "and from moment to moment integrates

its selection to give unity even to the most transient experiences"
(p. 362).

The argument is buttressed by neurophysiological data and contains many specific proposals, including one that the "readiness potential," which preceeds voluntary motor activity, is a marker of
the mind's effect on the brain. (We will return to the topic of the
readiness potential in the chapter on the polarity of conscious and
unconscious.) The means by which the mind exerts its actions on
the brain is not clearly stated, though the locus of that action is:

> Presumably the self-conscious mind does not act on the cortical modules
> with some bash operation, but rather with a slight deviation. A very
> gentle deviation up or down is all that is required. It may be conjec-
> tured that this effect builds up at the superficial laminae (I and II) and
> modulates and controls the discharges of pyramidal cells. . . . Further-
> more we would conjecture that the self-conscious mind is weak relative
> to the power of the synaptic mechanisms in laminae III, IV and V that
> are activated by the thalamic inputs. It is simply a deviator, and modi-
> fies the modular activity by its slight deviations. (Pp. 368–69)

As to the location and composition of the mind itself, Eccles is
vague. In his view, it is likely to have fundamentally different properties from those found in the physical realm, and "though it is in
liaison with special zones of the neocortex, it need not itself have
the property of spatial extention. . . . But the question: where is the
self-conscious mind located? is unanswerable in principle" (p. 376).

If the location of the mind cannot be known *in principle*, then
it seems that Eccles, despite his desire to propose refutable conjectures, has provided an essentialist explanation. To say that "it
makes no sense to ask where are located the feelings of love or hate,
or of joy or fear, or of such values as truth, goodness and beauty"
(p. 376) is to avoid, rather than satisfy, the gravamen of the materialist challenge to all dualistic arguments: *Where* is the mind?
*What* is it made of ? *How* does it work? A materialist does not worry
about unextended entities and insubstantial substances nor about
violating the first law of thermodynamics; for a materialist, feelings
and values are located in the brains of individuals who think them.

Indeed, in the opinion of some materialists, a brain as such is
not required in order to generate mental experiences. For many
working in the field of artificial intelligence, a computer, if properly
programmed, could be said to have thoughts, moods, and self-aware-
ness. [20] In this view, it does not matter what the "hardware" is made
of, so long as it simulates human thought.

But are computer-simulated "mental experiences" identical with human mental experiences? John Searle does not think so:

The idea that computer simulations could be the real thing ought to have seemed suspicious in the first place because the computer isn't confined to simulating mental operations, by any means. No one supposes that computer simulations of a five-alarm fire will burn the neighborhood down or that a computer simulation of a rainstorm will leave us all drenched. Why on earth would anyone suppose that a computer simulation of understanding actually understood anything? It is sometimes said that it would be frightfully hard to get computers to feel pain or fall in love, but love and pain are neither harder nor easier than cognition or anything else. For simulation, all you need is the right input and output and a program in the middle that transforms the former into the latter. That is all the computer has for anything it does. To confuse simulation with duplication is the same mistake, whether it is pain, love, cognition, fires, or rainstorms.[21]

Searle's views on the difference between simulation and duplication raise once again the problem all materialist theories face with regard to the mind-brain polarity: How are the physical events of the brain (or the computer) translated into *experiences*? How do you get from circuits (whether neural or electronic) to indignation, or to whimsy?

Materialist assertions about the eventual resolution of the mind-brain polarity do not account for the phenomenal world and the unity of conscious experience. They only promise to do so. We hold the opinion so well expressed by David Bakan:

Divergence between science and theory, on the one hand, and the universe of empirical observation, on the other hand, may speak to either a defect of science and theory, or a defect of empirical observation, or both. I do not derogate science and theory generally. Nonetheless, scientists and theorists must be able to offer powerful and cogent arguments if they ask that the results of experience and observation be dismissed as illusion.[22]

## Thinking in Terms of Psychiatric Methodology

The perspective of mind and the perspective of brain are both valid for a consideration of grief. But since they make different assumptions about human nature, we find, as we switch from one viewpoint to the other, that sometimes we see ourselves as subject/agents and at other times as object/organisms. Try as we might to hold both perspectives in focus—to adopt Baruch (Benedict De) Spinoza's position that Nature is an indivisible whole and that "substance thinking [mind] and substance extended [body] are one and the same substance, comprehended now through one attribute, now through the other"[23]—we find it most difficult to accomplish. Like the physicists who see light now as a particle, now as a wave, psychiatrists shift their viewpoint on the phenomenal world back and forth between the perspective of mind and the perspective of brain.

GRIEF AND THE BRAIN

If grief is to be explained as a process in the brain, as a reaction of object/organisms, then two fundamental questions (among others) must be answered: What is the biological basis of emotion? How is the experience of loss translated into the physiological expression of grief? Although neither issue has been resolved, promising work is in progress.

The first recorded proposal for the biological basis of emotions is found in the Hippocratic writings of the fourth century B.C., which related temperamental types and diseases to the preponderance of one or another bodily humor. Thus, the melancholic temperament and the disease "melancholia" were due to an excess of black bile.

This linking of normal and disordered emotions in a common biological substrate was the achievement of medicine because physicians, unlike nonclinical observers, were able to correlate mental disturbance with bodily pathology, to document emotional changes in patients whose brains had been injured in particular ways. Until this century, only such clinicopathological methods were available to study directly the relationship between mental life and brain processes in human beings. Since Hans Berger's discovery of the electro-encephalogram in 1929, however, techniques have been developed to enable investigators from both the clinical and the basic sciences to observe the intact brain and to correlate its activities with the experience and expression of emotion.

Still, much of what is known about the neural basis of emotion is derived from the work of physicians at the bedside, in the laboratory, and at the autopsy table. At the end of the nineteenth century the importance of subcortical brain mechanisms for the expression of emotion had been demonstrated, but it was not until the first decades of this century that the role of cortical structures in the experience of emotion had been shown. James Papez, for example, proposed in 1937 a neural apparatus for the integration of cortical and subcortical structures into a "harmonious mechanism" that both permitted the experience of emotion and participated in its expression.[24]

More recently, a cerebral lateralization of emotion has been suggested. Support for this hypothesis, which is based in part on studies of brain-injured patients and of those with psychiatric disorders, has been summarized by Pierre Flor-Henry, who maintains that "sadness is a function of right brain systems and euphoria of left brain systems."[25] Conjectures of this sort can be tested empirically, but in doing so, investigators cannot fully employ a standard research method: the use of animal subjects.

Although it is reasonable to extrapolate from certain animal behaviors to emotional states in humans, the inability of other animals to tell us of their experiences has made suitable research paradigms difficult to develop, not only for work on the neural basis of emotions but also for investigations into the relationship between loss and the physiology of grief. Despite this obstacle, however, much has been learned from the study of other species.

The separation of an infant from its mother provokes a response in the child that has been likened to the grief reaction seen in adults who have lost a beloved person.[26] The effects of early maternal separation cannot be studied experimentally in humans, but work with monkeys and rats has suggested that behavioral and physiological reactions to early maternal separation are a basic mammalian characteristic.[27]

Both grief reactions and separation reactions can be seen as wholes, as circumscribed episodes in the life of the animal. But these reactions can also be divided into phases that, though not always sharply demarcated from one another, show a predominance of certain sets of phenomena. With animal subjects, alterations in the phenomena of a given phase (e.g., activity levels, feeding, sleeping, cardiovascular functions) can be correlated with particular interventions (e.g., the return of the mother or the provision of a surrogate). In this way, the relationship between a type of loss and the physiology of emotional distress can be studied.

The work of Myron Hofer illustrates this line of investigation (pp. 245–64). Using two-week-old rat pups, he demonstrated that the absence of the mother elicited a pattern of behavioral hyperactivity comparable to the "protest" phase of the separation reaction in human children described by Bowlby. Across mammalian species, then, there seems to be an intrinsic behavioral response to maternal separation whose goal is to reunite the infant with its parent. The state of behavioral arousal experimentally produced in rat pups could be diminished by tactile and olfactory stimulation of the type usually provided by their mothers. What appeared to be essential in the reversal of hyperactivity was not maternal contact of any type but rather particular stimuli mediated by specific neural systems. In this work we have a model for explaining the biological substrate of attachment, dependency, and separation anxiety: psychological concepts related to the phenomenon of grief.

GRIEF AND THE MIND

For attempts to explain grief as a process in the brain, there are more questions than answers. For attempts to understand grief as a process in the mind, there are more answers than questions. This difference between the perspectives rests on the methods employed.

If "brain" proposals are true conjectures rather than essentialist explanations, they are set forth as hypotheses to be tested by empirical means; those that survive the tests are accepted (at least until the next round of testing), those that do not are discarded. But "mind" proposals usually cannot be winnowed in this way, since what they set forth is in the language of meaning. Thus, for example, psychoanalysis, existential philosophy, and religion all have contributions to make to our understanding of grief and mourning. These different viewpoints are not to be pitted against one another as hypotheses to be tested; rather, they are to be appreciated for the way in which each can illuminate a different aspect of the mourner's phenomenal world.

Because human relationships have meanings that cannot be conveyed by the language of biology, and because death has a significance beyond the physiology of grief, much of the experience and behavior of mourners is shaped by cultural forces. Here, the perspective of anthropology is helpful. In some societies, grief is expressed in a very emotional way, with wailing, the rending of clothes, and even with ritual self-mutilation.[28] Among other peoples, however, grief is emotionally constrained: Clifford Geertz observed of Javanese death customs that tears "are not approved of and certainly not encouraged. . . . *Iklas*, that state of willed affectlessness, is the watchword, and although it is often difficult to achieve, it is always striven for."[29]

Such differences in the expression of grief are not rooted in biological processes but in the concepts and customs of societies. The mourners are subject/agents, participants in a culture whose views on the meaning of life and death they have come to learn and helped to modify. Certain expressions (and the experiences that accompany them) are deemed proper, while others are considered abhorrent. The choice is not made for evolutionary advantage but to express, in symbolic form, the values of a people. Thus, to understand grief as a mental process, it is not only necessary to appreciate the significance of love and loss in individual terms, but also to see that life and death are collective experiences whose meanings are part of the consciousness of cultures.

## Conclusion

The polarity of mind and brain, here illustrated by the state of grief, seems intractable. No matter how much we learn about the brain, its links to the phenomenal world remain mysterious. Though we can sometimes *correlate* the occurrence of mental events with brain events, the *transformation* of neural processes into mental states (or vice versa) is unexplained. If there is to be a scientific accounting of the phenomenal world, it must reveal not only the material underpinnings of that world but also how it comes to be *experienced*.

To obliterate the gap between "mind" and "brain" will therefore demand something more than the identification of neural systems and the description of their functional relationships to one another. If science eventually explains how the brain can generate that unity of conscious experience we call the self and its phenomenal world, it will do so in terms we cannot imagine today. The resolution of the mind-brain polarity does not rest on current theories and technologies, but rather awaits the development of a revolutionary conception of human biology.

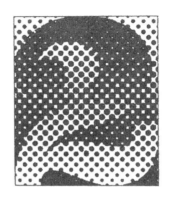

# Attempting to Deal with Ambiguity

# 3
# Explanation & Understanding

Because mental life is more than the sum of neural events, describing a brain and its functions is not the same thing as describing a self and its predicaments. Human beings exist in a world of meaning as well as in a world of matter, so that, as we shall see in this chapter, both the methods of the humanities and the methods of the natural sciences are essential to psychiatric practice.

## Manic-Depressive Illness

THE CASE OF VIRGINIA WOOLF

When studying English literature at university, we were taught that Virginia Woolf killed herself in 1941 because she could not face the cruelty and destruction of another World War. We learned that she had been not only a very talented person but also a painfully sensitive one, and that her mental illness and suicide attempts were due to the impact of devastating events on an artistic sensibility. This narrative way of appreciating Virginia Woolf's troubles seemed a most natural one, for we found that, through empathy, we could understand her suffering, if not her genius.

Several of Virginia Woolf's biographers have taken this approach to her illness and suicide. Anne Olivier Bell, for example, wrote that, while most of Virginia Woolf's childhood had been happy and secure, her mother's death in 1895 "was the end of all security and most happiness. The shock drove Virginia out of her mind."[1]

But it was not only death that could precipitate madness. As

Virginia's husband, Leonard Woolf, came to discover, the process of completing a novel was also something to be feared:

In January and February she was finishing *The Voyage Out,* writing every day with a kind of tortured intensity. I did not know then what over the years we learnt bitterly by experience, that the weeks or months in which she finished a book would always be a terrific mental and nervous strain upon her and bring her to the verge of a mental breakdown. It was not merely the strain of the mental intensity with which she always wrote, the artistic integrity and ruthlessness which made her drive herself remorselessly towards perfection. She also suffered from what most people would say was a weakness or fault of character, but which was intricately entangled with her mental instability, an almost pathological hypersensitiveness to criticism, so that she suffered an ever increasingly agonizing nervous apprehension as she got nearer and nearer to the end of her book and the throwing of it and of herself to the critics.[2]

Leonard Woolf saw this process at first hand and so was able to link certain traits of his wife's personality with events in her life and subsequent episodes of madness. But a more distant observer could also find such connections and could read in them not only the torment of Virginia Woolf, but also a kind of suffering common to many artists:

Almost anyone who has attempted to create a work of art will have an inkling of what she then felt. A book is so much a part of oneself that in delivering it to the public one feels as if one were pushing one's own child out into the traffic. If it be killed or hurt the injury is done to oneself, and if it be one's first-born, the product of seven years' gestation . . . needing all the tenderness and all the understanding that no critic will ever give, anxiety for its fate becomes acute.

Virginia already knew whither such anxieties might lead her. She knew that she had to be sensible and to exert self-control if the horrors of 1895 and 1904 and 1910 were not to be repeated. But . . . her sleepless nights were spent in wondering whether her art, the whole meaning and purpose of her life, was fatuous, whether it might not be torn to shreds by a discharge of cruel laughter.[3]

But despite our immediate empathic identification with such narratives, despite their sense of rightness, what was so convincing to students of English literature is not convincing enough to students of psychiatry. If anxiety about reviews is so common among artists, why are not more of them mad? Surely there must have been something about Virginia Woolf that made her more vulnerable, or vulnerable in a different way, to the stresses of the creative life. Besides, if upsetting events triggered episodes of insanity, why were not all of her losses (such as the death of her brother) and the publication of all of her novels followed by madness? And why did some of her attacks seem to occur unheralded by loss or worry? Indeed, what do such events have to do with *madness*—for that is what afflicted Virginia Woolf—rather than with grief or anxious procrastination? The particular *form* of her distress must be accounted for if we are to have an accurate understanding of Virginia Woolf's life and death.

There can be no doubt that Virginia Woolf suffered from manic-depressive disorder; she had an episodic illness characterized by changes in mood and self-attitude, with delusions, hallucinations, and disturbed sleep, appetite, and energy. Again, the acute observations of Leonard Woolf are of interest:

In all these cases of breakdown there were two distinct stages which are technically called manic-depressive. In the manic stage she was extremely excited; the mind raced; she talked volubly and, at the height of the attack, incoherently; she had delusions and heard voices, for instance she told me that in her second attack she heard the birds in the garden outside her window talking Greek; she was violent with the nurses. . . . During the depressive stage all her thoughts and emotions were the exact opposite of what they had been in the manic stage. She was in the depths of melancholia and despair; she scarcely spoke; refused to eat; refused to believe that she was ill and insisted that her condition was due to her own guilt; at the height of this stage she tried to commit suicide.[4]

Seen from the perspective of this devastating illness, another light is cast on her death. In a suicide note to her husband, Virginia Woolf wrote:

I feel certain that I am going mad again: I feel we cant go through another of those terrible times. And I shant recover this time. I begin to hear voices, and cant concentrate. So I am doing what seems to be the best thing to do. . . . I dont think two people could have been happier till this terrible disease came. I cant fight it any longer. . . . Everything has gone from me but the certainty of your goodness. I cant go on spoiling your life any longer.[5]

Here, as in the proposal that she killed herself because of the War, we understand *why*, but our understanding is very different this time. In the context of her illness we see, not a sensitive artist appalled at the destruction of civilization, but the victim of a disorder who has become demoralized in her struggle to overcome it. Thus it may be, as Quentin Bell observed:

To know that you have had a cancer in your body and to know that it may return must be very horrible; but a cancer of the mind, a corruption of the spirit striking one at the age of thirteen and for the rest of one's life always working away somewhere, always in suspense . . . this must be almost unendurable. So unendurable that in the end, when the voices of insanity spoke to her in 1941, she took the only remedy that remained, the cure of death.[6]

And yet the voices of insanity had spoken to Virginia Woolf before, and she had attempted to kill herself several times in the past. Thus, once again the fact of her manic-depressive disorder comes to the fore in our attempts to explain her mental illness and death. The disorder was characterized by auditory hallucinations and delusions of hopelessness and guilt. Though we can understand such phenomena as motives for suicide, their occurrence in the first place is mysterious. Had she not suffered from manic-depressive disorder, Virginia Woolf might not have died at the time or in the manner she did; indeed, had she not suffered from manic-depressive disorder she might not have written as she did:

After being ill and suffering every form and variety of nightmare and extravagant intensity of perception—for I used to make up poems, stories, profound and to me inspired phrases all day long as I lay in bed, and thus sketched, I think, all that I now, by the light of reason, try to put into prose (I thought of the Lighthouse then, and Kew and others, not in substance, but in idea)—after all this, when I came to, I was so tremblingly afraid of my own insanity that I wrote Night and Day mainly to prove to my own satisfaction that I could keep entirely off that dangerous ground.[7]

A METHODOLOGICAL OBSERVATION

As we study the illness of Virginia Woolf, we are continually aware of a tension between two views of mental disorder. In one, the phenomenal world of the patient is approached "from within," through the human capacity for empathy: we appreciate how one mental event grows out of another, and how the present is a development of the past. This appreciation takes the form of a narrative, a life story, in which the patient's distress is seen to emerge from an interaction between a self and a situation.

Here, too, we understand the *content* of mental experiences, that is, what the patient is anxious *about*, what the hallucinated voices *say*. Such matters can only be understood from our knowledge of the individual patient's life—her interests, relationships, cultural background and the like. From this perspective, the patient is seen as a *subject* or an *agent* rather than as an *object* or an *organism*. In this way we can appreciate not only why, in her illness of 1895, Virginia Woolf could have the experience that "King Edward VII lurked in the azaleas using the foulest possible language,"[8] but also that the content of her hallucinations and delusions would have been most unlikely had she grown up in Wisconsin and lived a century earlier.

In the other view of mental illness, the phenomenal world of the patient must be observed "from without," because empathic understanding fails to account for the *form* of the illness and the relentless course it takes. Thus, while the content of Virginia Woolf's hallucinations might be understood, at least in part, from her Victorian childhood, the fact that she was *hallucinating* cannot. The explanation of how Virginia Woolf, or anyone else, can experience hallucinations (i.e., perceptions without stimuli) is a mystery, though we can correlate the occurrence of hallucinations with certain types of known brain disease and with psychiatric syndromes for which the disease concept seems an appropriate model.[9] To explain the form of disorder, we must rely, not on empathy, but on the methods of the natural sciences, and we tend to see the patient more as an object/organism than as a subject/agent.

As we noted in *The Perspectives of Psychiatry* (pp. 11–26), these views of mental illness constitute a dialectic in which there is thesis and antithesis, but no synthesis. When we direct our attention to the content of the disorder and its illumination through the method of empathy, we tend to overlook the fact that some illnesses arise from damaged brains and thus can affect large numbers of very different people in exactly the same way. And when we concentrate on the form of the disorder and its elucidation through the methods of the natural sciences, we tend to miss the meaning of the illness for the patient and the clues it offers to his unique life story. These two ways of approaching mental illness rest on fundamentally different methods of reaꞏ ꞏning—on the polarity of *explanation* and *understanding*.

## The Polarity of Explanation and Understanding

HISTORY

The polarity of explanation and understanding has its roots deep in the history of science, in a tension between two traditions that Georg Henrik von Wright termed the *aristotelian* and the *galilean*.[10] The aristotelian view of science is teleological in nature and seeks to understand the ends of things. The galilean view, on the other hand, is causal and mechanistic in character and has as its goal the prediction of phenomena.

In the ninteenth century, the contrast between these two traditions was seen in a new guise, as historians and other social scientists tried to defend the interpretative, aristotelian methods of their disciplines against the attacks of positivist critics, who held that valid knowledge could be derived only from the galilean methods of the natural sciences. The claims for interpretation were based on the observation that the world of human beings is radically different from the nonhuman world and that it must therefore be approached in a fundamentally different way. As Max Wartofsky and Richard Zaner note in their review of this conflict, in the positivist

approach to the nature of scientific knowledge, the term *Erklären* (explaining) was used to designate the primarily causal explanations taken to be characteristic of the natural sciences, and of physics in particular. It connoted, further, that the phenomena studied in this way were lawlike (nomological), that is, that there were universal, or at least general, laws or patterns in terms of which individual cases could be accounted for, or taken as instances of these laws. The force of this type of view is that, knowing the lawlike character or the causal structure of a domain, one could predict a given case or the course of an individual event, once its antecedent conditions were sufficiently known. . . . The form of such causal or lawlike structures could then be represented in logical or mathematical terms, such that predictions followed deductively from lawlike statements. . . .

By contrast . . . methodologists of the social sciences argued that human activity could not be understood in such a manner, that distinctively human actions were not lawlike or causal in the specific sense in which these terms and their cognates applied to physical nature. Rather, human phenomena generally could be understood properly only in terms of what it is that agents of such actions themselves believed that they were doing or intended to do. Thus . . . to understand a human action requires that one understand the way or ways in which the agent of the action himself understands and interprets his own action; its "meaning" is the meaning it has for the agent whose action it is. Beliefs and intentions, unlike natural phenomena, connote the conscious activity of agents subject to their own free (or relatively free) choice, or at least to their own self-comprehension. If there are lawlike patterns in such behavior, thus, it was said to be describable in terms of rules rather than laws, and to be accounted for in terms of reasons rather than causes. The kind of understanding to be achieved here . . . was distinguished from *Erklären* (explaining) and was designated *Verstehen* (understanding).[11]

INTRODUCTION INTO PSYCHIATRY

The polarity of explanation and understanding was introduced into psychiatry by Karl Jaspers. Unlike Johann Gustav Droysen, Wilhelm Dilthey, Max Weber, and the other social scientists who had developed and defended the concept of *Verstehen*, Jaspers was a physician. For him there could be no choice between explanation and understanding, since his patients were both agents *and* organisms, subjects *and* objects—since they had both minds *and* brains. The issue for Jaspers was, therefore, not which method was the correct approach to psychiatry, but rather which was the most useful in a given set of circumstances.

As a phenomenologist, Jaspers was interested in the nature of events in the phenomenal world and, as well, in the connections between them, in both observation and interpretation. In some cases, the connections are immediately apparent, and through *Verstehen* ("perception of meaning") we can understand

directly *how one psychic event emerges from another*. This mode of understanding is only possible with psychic events. In this way we can be said to understand the anger of someone attacked, the jealousy of the man made cuckold, the acts and decisions that spring from motive.[12]

In other cases, however, such as the occurrence of psychotic phenomena (e.g., hallucinations) or the loss of psychological capacities (e.g., aphasia), psychiatrists must rely on *Erklären* ("perception of causal connection"), since

understanding (or perception of meaningful connection) soon reaches its *limits*. . . . In psychopathology psychic phenomena appear suddenly as something entirely new, in a way we cannot understand at all. One psychic event follows another quite incomprehensibly; it seems to follow arbitrarily rather than emerge. . . . We can only resort to *causal explanation*, as with phenomena in the natural sciences, which . . . are never seen "from within" but "from the outside" only. (Pp. 27–28)

According to Jaspers, this explaining "from the outside" is inescapable because causal connections have their foundations in the somatic realm, in biological phenomena that are themselves beyond the reach of consciousness and thus beyond the reach of understanding. In his view, causal connections can only be established empirically, by the hypothetico-deductive methods of the natural sciences, and can only be accounted for by a theory that links the phenomenal to the biological.

But how is the existence of meaningful connections established, and how can they be validated, if the procedures and criteria of the natural sciences are inappropriate? These questions lead us to a further consideration of the characteristics of *Verstehen*, which, we have found, are less familiar to students of psychiatry than are those of *Erklären*.

THE METHOD OF UNDERSTANDING

Jaspers distinguished between two modes of understanding (p. 27). In the first, which he termed *static*, the task of phenomenology is to determine the form of a mental event or state (e.g., that it is a thought rather than a perception; that it is a mood of anxiety rather than of elation). Here, the emphasis is on the *what* of the patient's mental experiences. In the second type of understanding, termed *genetic*, the effort is to appreciate the connectedness of psychic events, the emergence of one from another. Here, the psychiatrist uses his empathic and rational powers to grasp the *why* of the patient's thoughts, moods, and behaviors. It is this second type of *Verstehen* that speaks to the issue of meaning in mental life.

The existence and validation of meaningful connections reached through genetic understanding depends on criteria other than those of the natural sciences:

In the natural sciences we find causal connections *only* but in psychology our bent for knowledge is satisfied with the comprehension of quite a different sort of connection. Psychic events "emerge" out of each other in a way which we understand. Attacked people become angry and spring to the defence, cheated persons grow suspicious. . . .

This strikes us as something self-evident which cannot be broken down any further. . . . It carries its own power of conviction and it is a precondition of the psychology of meaningful phenomena that we accept this kind of evidence just as acceptance of the reality of perception and of causality is the precondition of the natural sciences. (Pp. 302–3)

But if genetic understanding rests on the conviction that something is self-evident, it does not follow that the method completely ignores the usual standards of scientific evidence:

The self-evidence of a meaningful connection does not prove that in a particular case that connection is *really there*. . . . In any given case the judgment of whether a meaningful connection is real does not rest on its self-evident character alone. It depends primarily *on the tangible facts* (that is, on the verbal contents, cultural factors, people's acts, ways of life, and expressive gestures) in terms of which the connection is understood, and which provide the objective data. All such objective data, however, are always incomplete and our understanding of *any particular, real event* has to remain more or less an *interpretation* which only in a few cases reaches any relatively high degree of complete and convincing objectivity. . . . The fewer these [objective data] are, the less forcefully do they compel our understanding; we interpret more and understand less. (P. 303)

That meaningful connections rest on an interpretation of empirical data is the first of six basic properties Jaspers attributed to the method of understanding. These characteristics form the standards by which the results of understanding can be evaluated, and it is to them that we now turn.

THE PROPERTIES OF MEANINGFUL CONNECTIONS

The first property of meaningful connections is that they are interpretations. Given the same set of objective data, our "psychological imagination . . . continually designs for us what seem to be convincing patterns as such, yet . . . another possible way of understanding is always at hand" (p. 356). This characteristic of meaningful connections is often seen in the vigorous disagreements that can occur during case conferences between discussants of different theoretical persuasions.

The second attribute of meaningful connections is that they follow "the hermeneutic round." By this Jaspers meant that the interpretation we give to an event in the patient's mental life is dependent to some extent on the concepts we already hold, and that once the interpretation is formed, it reaffirms and expands those concepts. Thus, we understand a patient's compulsions as the expression of a need for control, and the occurrence of those compulsions leads us to discover in his experiences and behavior other manifestations of that need.

The third property of meaningful connections is that opposite interpretations are equally convincing. We can understand, for example, that someone with a fear of heights is unlikely to climb mountains, but the opposite connection is equally meaningful—that someone fearful of heights becomes a mountaineer in order to overcome his phobia. Jaspers warned that

> the most radical mistakes spring from conclusions drawn as to the reality of what has been understood, whenever these conclusions have been based on the self-evidence of some one-sided understanding. The exclusion of the opposite, without any attempt to follow it up and understand it, means that we manipulate reality in favour of an "a priori" understanding that makes an arbitrary selection of the facts. (P. 357)

The fourth characteristic of meaningful connections is that they are inconclusive. In part, this is because they rest on interpretations, which may never acquire enough empirical support to convince us that all which could be known is known, and in part because they are rooted in biological mechanisms (such as instinctual drives), which cannot themselves be grasped through understanding. But meaningful connections are also inconclusive because life is happening as we observe and interpret it, and because the final chapter cannot be written for someone who has both choice and a future.

The fifth property of meaningful connections is that they are unlimited in number:

> As soon as we believe we can make some definite interpretation, another presents itself. . . . It lies in the very essence of meaningfulness. . . . On the other hand, as empirically accessible material grows, understanding becomes more decisive. Multiplicity does not necessarily imply haphazard uncertainty but can mean a flexible movement within the range of possibility that leads to an increasing certainty of vision. (Pp. 358–59)

Jaspers's sixth attribute of meaningful connections is that to understand is both to illuminate and to expose aspects of mental life. This double function is inherent in the method of understanding, though in practice he felt that a malevolent exposure of deceptions seems to predominate:

> In a mood of scepticism or dislike we think we are always "seeing through it." . . . There is a mischievous psychology of opposites in which opposites are used simply to turn all that an individual does, says or wants into the opposite of what seems to be his real meaning. Symbolic interpretation is brought into use in order to find the meaning of every

drive in some unconscious baseness that has been repressed. . . . In contrast to this, understanding which illuminates and does not expose involves an attitude which is basically positive. It approaches human nature sympathetically. (P. 359)

To these six Jasperian properties of meaningful connections we can add another, one that is characteristic of them when they are presented as general facts of human nature.[13] In this form, meaningful connections that were seen in the lives of a few patients are held to play important roles in the lives of many. Thus we have Josef Breuer and Sigmund Freud's claim that *"Hysterics suffer mainly from reminiscences,"*[14] and Harry Stack Sullivan's dictum that "The hysteric might be said in principle to be a person who has a happy thought as to a way by which he can be respectable even though not living up to his standards."[15] Such meaningful connections are often treated as if they were laws, whereas in truth they are more like maxims or proverbs (e.g., "Absence makes the heart grow fonder."). They do not find their use in the prediction of thoughts and behaviors but rather in making sense of what has already occurred.

As a physician and a philosopher, Jaspers appreciated that these properties of understanding could make the method seem irritatingly "soft," but he was at pains to remind his readers that the realm of meaning is real and that it must be taken on its own terms:

Understanding . . . in defining the knowledge it is aiming at, must not adopt the orientation of the natural sciences nor use their criteria nor must it take over the formal logic of mathematics. The truth which understanding seeks has other criteria, such as vividness, connectedness, depth and complexity.[16]

## Thinking in Terms of Psychiatric Methodology

Psychiatry's domain is the phenomenal world, something that must be explained *and* understood. If there were no gap between mind and brain, if meaningful connections were identical with neuronal connections, the method of explanation would be all that was required for psychiatric practice. Such is not the case. Selves are more than brains, and the method of understanding is needed to discover their intentions, appreciate their emotions, interpret their beliefs, and see their predicaments.

Explanation and understanding are thus basic concepts in psychiatric methodology. As you read further in this book you will see their implications in other polarities, and should you review the lively debate over the scientific status of psychoanalysis, you will appreciate their significance to theorists and philosophers. Yet despite their importance in psychiatric reasoning, the concepts of explanation and understanding are seldom discussed in the field. Perhaps this is because methodological issues are thought to be trivial pursuits or because it is believed they have already been resolved (at least in principle), but whatever the reasons, the cost of our neglect has been substantial.

As noted above, psychiatrists may confuse the maxims of understanding with the laws of explanation. This is dangerous because the sense of conviction generated by meaningful connections is often a powerful one, so that what are no more than opinions and hunches may be presented as facts of human nature or as prescriptions for the well-being of society. And because these opinions and hunches are proposed with confidence and good intentions, psychiatrists may not notice that they are supported by little more than their plausibility. The result of this unreflective enthusiasm is that the meaningful claims of psychiatry have often been oversold, and as a consequence the public has understandably questioned the validity and value of our work as a whole.

But if understanding is sometimes accorded a scope it does not deserve, it is also denied a status it clearly merits. Some psychiatrists act as if explanation were the only legitimate method for physicians to use and treat understanding as if it were merely "common sense," rather than a concept that has engaged profound students of psychiatry, psychology, and philosophy; as if it were something to help the "worried well," rather than the basis of what might be life-saving therapeutic work in the care of the distressed and the demoralized.

Our lack of knowledge about the assumptions and consequences of explanation and understanding has also been an important reason for the enervating and embarrassing squabbles that erupt over questions like, "Is the fundamental problem in hysteria related to sex, as Freud held, or to insecurity, as Sullivan claimed?" (Answer: "There is no 'fundamental' problem where understanding is concerned, because interpretation is unlimited and incomplete. Try to learn a variety of meaningful theories so that you can use the one that best fits your patient and your goals.") and "Who are the *real* psychiatrists?" (Answer: "That's the wrong question. It would be better to ask about the nature of various mental disorders and how they should be comprehended and treated. All psychiatrists are real psychiatrists.")

THE CASE OF VIRGINIA WOOLF

In the case of Virginia Woolf the complementary nature of explanation and understanding can be seen. We must be clear, however, about the indications for reasoning from one method rather than the other as we seek to illuminate different aspects of her illness. The fact of Virginia Woolf's manic-depressive disorder, for example, seems mostly a matter for explanation.

We do not mean here that, given the present state of knowledge, we can explain how Virginia Woolf came to have manic-depressive disorder, nor do we mean that understandable factors had no role in the onset or resolution of her attacks, but we do mean that the disorder itself, the *fact* of it as an occurrence in Nature, is something that needs explanation.

Manic-depressive disorder is a clinical syndrome for which the disease concept is an appropriate mode of reasoning.[17] Its form (that of an episodic illness characterized by a primary change in mood and self-attitude, accompanied by disturbances in sleep, appetite, and well-being, and often by delusions and hallucinations) is not only distinctive but also quite similar from patient to patient, culture to culture, and epoch to epoch. As well, the syndrome has been observed to occur as part of known diseases of the brain (such as Huntington's disease) and to have a genetic transmission in some families (linked, for example, to a gene on the X-chromosome). Such features, when added to the regularity and universality of manic-depressive disorder, suggest that it is grounded in abnormal human biology, and thus that the discovery of its cause is a matter for the disciplines of genetics, neuroscience, and epidemiology—for the methods of explanation.

Not only did Virginia Woolf have manic-depressive disorder; she also tried repeatedly to kill herself. How should we reason about her suicide? Though we will return to the topic of suicide in the chapter on the polarity of autonomy and paternalism, we might begin here by appreciating that suicide is a behavior (pp.101–4). Like other behaviors, such as drug abuse and the food refusal of anorexia nervosa, suicide is an act defined by its goals—in this case, the taking of one's life. Virginia Woolf's suicidal behavior occured only when she manifested other signs of manic-depressive disorder (such as delusions of guilt or hopelessness), and thus, in a crucial way, her death by suicide is something to be explained, for the fact of manic-depressive disorder is something to be explained.

But suicide, like other behaviors, has multiple determinants, and some of those determinants are best viewed from the perspective of the individual as subject/agent rather than as object/organism. One must *choose* to take one's life, and even in manic-depressive disorder, where the risk of suicide is much higher than in the general population, not everyone makes that choice. Thus, in the case of Virginia Woolf, we can ask, as we ask with all suicides, "Why?" When we seek to discover the reasons for her behavior, when we try to link her final act with the life that went before it, we have entered the realm of understanding.

From the perspective of understanding, Virginia Woolf's suicide is seen as the final chapter in her life story, a story that includes manic-depressive illness, but much else besides. In life-story reasoning,[18] we try to appreciate a person rather than to explain a syndrome. Here, suicide is not only the symptom of a disorder but also the choice of a self, and it is characteristic of life-story reasoning that the choice comes to be viewed as the meaningful outcome of all that went before. Thus, in the life story of Virginia Woolf as told by Quentin Bell, her suicide was interpreted as "the only remedy that remained."

LEVELS OF UNDERSTANDING

Our understanding of Virginia Woolf's suicide can be said to occur at three levels, the first of which is based on meaningful connections within her phenomenal world. As recorded in her suicide note, Virginia Woolf was demoralized and hopeless about her illness and guilty about its effects on the life of her husband. These ideas were delusional in nature: though she had been ill and recovered several times in the past (having been prevented from taking her life), she nonetheless believed that all had been lost and thus that suicide was "the best thing to do." Given Virginia Woolf's perception of the world, we can understand in an empathic way the choice she made. Though her assumptions were false, once they are accepted, the reasoning behind her suicide seems logical and its motivation meaningful. Here the method of understanding places us "within" Virginia Woolf's phenomenal world, helps us see life through her eyes, and demonstrates how one psychic event can grow out of another.

At a second level of understanding, meaningful connections link the phenomenal world of Virginia Woolf to what we know of her life. In this way we can appreciate that the death of her mother was a painful loss and that it could precipitate the onset of a disorder to which she was vulnerable on other grounds. Once that illness began, Virginia Woolf's suicidal behavior can be understood "from within." (It is important to remember here that understanding would lead us to expect a grief reaction at the death of a parent; the occurrence of manic-depressive disorder under these circumstances seems to be a matter for explanation.)

At the final level of understanding, the meaningful connections made may have more to do with those who employ the method than with the individual being understood. When we have neither a detailed description of the patient's phenomenal world, nor an authoritative knowledge of the events in her life, we rely on our capacity for empathy, on culturally determined views about the logic of certain behaviors, and on our acquaintance with meaningful theories (including those that propose unconscious motivations and conflicts) to help close the gaps in our understanding. In this way, we "uncover" plausible and convincing themes in the patient's life story that help us make sense of her actions. For example, given that Virginia Woolf was a sensitive person who had been appalled by World War I, what could be more "natural" than to understand her suicide as an act precipitated by a war that promised even more death and devastation than the last? In the process of constructing a life story for someone like Virginia Woolf, we may be captivated by the appeal of what has been termed "narrative truth"[19] and, almost without realizing it, give up the search for "historical truth."

As more information has become available about Virginia Woolf, it is clear that thoughts of the War did not play a large role (or even any role) in her suicide. In fact, just days before her death she wrote:

Still, I agree that this war's better than last, and ever so much better than the last 5 years of peace. We've been bombed out of London and live entirely here now. Leonard lectures the village on politics. We see Vanessa occasionally—most nights the raiders go over. Last week the haystacks blazed and incendiaries lit up the downs. I cant help wishing the invasion would come. Its this standing about in a dentist's waiting room that I hate.[20]

Our teachers at the university almost certainly had no knowledge of this letter or of Virginia Woolf's suicide note when they taught us that she had taken her life because of the War. Like clinicians, they used the information at hand to make sense of what had occurred. Theirs was a historical task, and the method of understanding provided a satisfying answer to the question: "Why did Virginia Woolf kill herself?"

But in the clinical setting, understanding has more than a historical function. The conclusions it produces not only give coherence to the past in the form of a life story, they also contribute to a psychotherapeutic process whose purpose is to change the future. As we will see in the chapter on the polarity of *Hebraic* and *Hellenic*, the effectiveness of psychotherapy depends more on the relationship established between the therapist and the patient than it does on the information they exchange. The method of understanding enhances the psychotherapeutic relationship because it provides a meaningful context for a shared human endeavor.

## Conclusion

The methods of explanation and understanding are both formal modes of reasoning in psychiatry. Though they have different assumptions about and consequences for our views on mental life, they stand on equal footing and in a complementary relationship to one another. We will emphasize explanation or understanding, depending on whether the issue is one of form or content, mechanism or meaning, brain or mind. This choice must be made knowingly rather than simply because we find one method more appealing. Explanation is no more "fundamental" than understanding, nor is understanding more "profound" than explanation; they are only different methods, with different strengths and weaknesses. As long as we continue to view human beings as object/organisms *and* subject/agents, both methods are essential to our practice.

# 4
# Conscious
# & Unconscious

Although some events in the phenomenal world can be explained through the methods of the natural sciences and others understood through the methods of the humanities, many experiences and behaviors remain mysterious as to their origins and persistence. In this chapter, we will explore a polarity that has developed in response to that mystery.

## Pseudoseizures

THE CASE OF MR. B.

Mr. B. was a 25-year-old single male who had been admitted for evaluation of seizurelike spells of three weeks duration.

*Family History:* The patient's father, a 49-year-old high school graduate and carpenter, was in good health. Mr. B. described him as a quiet, perfectionistic, hard-working, and dignified man who was made uncomfortable by displays of emotion. The patient and his father had always had a good, if distant, relationship, though Mr. B. felt he had never fully gained his father's approval. His mother, a 47-year-old high school graduate and homemaker, had a history of insulin-dependent diabetes mellitus. Mr. B. described her as an intelligent and affectionate woman to whom he felt very close, but also noted that, while he was growing up, she had to spend a great deal of time caring for his epileptic brother—something he often resented.

The patient's brother (his only sibling), was 23 years old, single, and living at home. The brother had suffered perinatal anoxia and developed generalized seizures as a child. His epilepsy had been difficult to control, and the family's plans often had to be changed because of his ill health. Despite frequent absences from school, the brother had been a good student and had graduated from a local college with a degree in accounting. As the brother grew out of adolescence his seizures lessened in frequency, and now he suffered only one or two per year, which did not interfere with his job in an insurance company. The patient described his brother as having been spoiled as a child, and though he respected him for having dealt successfully with a serious illness, Mr. B. often remembered having been jealous of his brother because the latter received a great deal of attention from their parents.

There was no other family history of epilepsy and none of psychiatric disorder.

*Personal History:* The patient's gestation, birth, and early development were uncomplicated. His health as a child was generally good, save for the usual childhood diseases, a tonsillectomy at age five years, and a concussion at age 11 years. The concussion occurred when the patient was accidentally struck in the head with a baseball bat during a game. After the blow Mr. B. was unconscious for several minutes and had to be admitted to the hospital overnight for observation. There were no sequelae of the injury except for several days of left frontotemporal headaches, which caused the patient to stay home from school. (He remembered this incident as one of the few times he had ever received more attention than his brother did.)

Mr. B. started school at age five, and graduated from high school at age 18. He was an average scholar and got on well with his teachers and classmates, though he did not participate in extracurricular activities because he had to work in a supermarket for spending money. (The patient recalled that he had been resentful of this because his brother, who did not work, had received an allowance.)

After graduation from high school, Mr. B. decided to work fulltime at the supermarket rather than to attend college because he wanted to be on his own. He progressed from stock boy to checker to assistant section manager over five years, but he was worried about his future because of rumors that the supermarket chain was not doing well and might have to close several branches.

The patient learned about sexual matters in a health course in junior high school. (His said his father was "too inhibited" to talk of such things.) Mr. B. began to date in the ninth grade and had several girlfriends, though no steady relationship until two years before admission, when he met his fiancée. She was now 22 years old and a teller at the bank across the street from the patient's place of employment. He described her as a serious and affectionate person who enjoyed reading and cooking. They had been sexually intimate several times, and both had found this part of their relationship entirely satisfactory.

Six months prior to the patient's admission to the hospital the couple had decided to marry but had not set a date because their financial situation was unclear. The patient's fiancée had urged him to study electronics or computer programming, since these occupations would offer more security and better pay than the supermarket might. This would be important to them because she wanted to begin a family as soon as possible. They quarreled over these matters, and several weeks prior to the patient's admission, during a heated argument, his fiancée threatened to break off their engagement.

The patient's health as an adult had been good. He drank alcohol in moderation but did not smoke or use illicit drugs.

*Premorbid Personality:* Mr. B. described his personality as that of a quiet man who was meticulous in his appearance and habits. He said that sometimes he had trouble expressing his feelings, but people should not assume he had none.

The patient's mother described him as a neat, moody, and somewhat introverted person. She noted that he had been jealous of his brother and that, when she tried to talk to him about his feelings, he tended to become sulky and withdrawn.

*Medical History:* None, save as noted above.

*Previous Psychiatric History:* None.

*History of the Present Illness:* The patient was in his usual state of good health until three weeks prior to admission when, during a quarrel with his fiancée, he had his first "seizure." His fiancée reported that Mr. B. was very angry at the time and stood before her with clenched fists and reddened face. He raised his hand as if to strike her but then began to "shake all over." He slumped to the ground and, with eyes tightly closed, began to have jerking movements of his arms and legs. After a few moments he stopped moving, opened his eyes, and asked what had happened. He had not been cyanotic, nor had he injured himself or been incontinent. He complained of a headache but did not seem confused. His fiancée notified his parents and then drove him to the emergency room, where they were met by his mother.

Neurological examination in the emergency room was normal, as it was when the patient was seen at a neurologist's office the next morning. EEG and CT scans of the head were also normal three days later. Despite reassurance that he probably had not had an epileptic seizure, in the following weeks the patient had three more spells, all much like the first in character. The second episode also occurred during a quarrel with his fiancée, the other two during visits with his parents.

One week before admission to the psychiatry service the patient was admitted to neurology, where a repeat EEG (sleep-deprived) was normal. A video-EEG was obtained with saline injection and the suggestion that the patient might have a seizure, which he did. At this time Mr. B. was noted to have the gradual onset (without cry or apparent aura) of tonic-clonic movements of all his limbs. This lasted some two minutes, during which the patient resisted attempts to open his eyes. He was breathing heavily, but there was no cyanosis, incontinence, tongue biting, or postictal confusion. Plantar responses were flexor. The EEG was normal, as was serum prolactin drawn 20 minutes after the spell.

Later that day the patient's neurologist told him the "seizures" were not epileptic in nature but were of the type precipitated by emotional distress, and that a psychiatric consultation was indicated. At first the patient refused, stating he knew his spells were not imaginary, but after reassurance that the fact of the spells was not in question, but rather their cause, he agreed.

*Mental Status Examination:* The patient was a neatly groomed, alert, perfectly oriented, and cooperative young man who made good eye contact. There were no abnormalities of movement, obvious hallucinations, or apparent seizures. He spoke a moderate amount, both spontaneously and in reply to questions. Speech was prompt, full, and without evidence of thought disorder. Mood was described as "worried" and appeared slightly apprehensive. Delusions, hallucinations, suicidal thoughts, obsessions, compulsions, and phobias were denied. Cognitive functions were intact.

Although at first Mr. B. denied that anything was troubling him except his spells, he soon acknowledged that he was worried about the future of both his engagement and his job. Though he could not see how such concerns might be linked to his illness, the patient agreed to an inpatient evaluation on psychiatry because he did not want the spells to get out of hand, as had happened to his brother.

*Treatment and Course:* Over the next several days the patient talked more freely of his spells. Although he could not explain how the first one had happened, he said that, at the time, he was very angry because he was "sick and tired" of always having to defer to someone else's needs. After the spell Mr. B. had been touched by the concern his fiancée and mother had shown and remembered thinking that, in his family, "you only get made a fuss over when you're sick." Each of the subsequent spells occurred when the patient was angry and had difficulty expressing his emotions. He "kind of knew" he was going to "lose control" and let himself do so.

Brief insight-oriented psychotherapy focused on issues and relationships, both past and present, that had upset Mr. B., and assertiveness training helped him express his feelings more appropriately. He was discharged to outpatient care after two weeks and, at follow-up six months later, had had no further spells.

THE ISSUE

How should we interpret the patient's pseudoseizures? On the one hand, his behavior could be the expression of an unconscious conflict or need, and therefore be termed a *conversion reaction*. On the other hand, it could be the manifestation of a conscious intention to produce certain responses in those around him, and therefore be termed *malingering*. Do the pseudoseizures represent a process hidden from the patient, or something he tries to hide from us? Pseudoseizures, like other "hysterical" phenomena, raise the issue of the polarity of conscious and unconscious.

## The Polarity of Conscious and Unconscious

When thinking as lay people rather than as psychiatrists, we clearly understand the meanings of the terms *conscious* and *unconscious*. We apply the former, for instance, to being awake and the latter to being asleep. But we also know that the terms are used in another way. People are said to be conscious or unconscious *of* something, in the sense of being aware or unaware of it. And just as we can illustrate the first usage of the terms by the difference between being awake and being asleep, so, too, we can draw on our own experiences to illustrate the second. When learning to drive an automobile, for example, we are very *self*-conscious as we think through what must be done and whether or not we are doing it correctly—all the while being very aware of our sense of uncertainty, our desire not to embarrass ourselves, and the way we might feel if admonished by the instructor. With enough practice, however, we become conscious of the fact that we can drive "without thinking about it" because the act of driving has become "automatic"; it is now something we do "unconsciously."

If these were the only senses in which the words were used, relatively little controversy would attend them. But because *conscious* and *unconscious* have been given other meanings by psychiatrists and psychologists, their nature and relationship have been hotly debated. For both terms two basic questions can be asked: Does the phenomenon exist? And if so, how should it be characterized?

IN DEFENSE OF CONSCIOUS

To question the existence of consciousness seems, at first, ridiculous. We could not be writing this, nor you reading it, unless we were all conscious. Indeed, to use the words *we* and *you* for selves thinking about something presupposes that we are conscious beings. This relationship between consciousness, thought, and personal identity has exercised philosophers, physicians, and scientists for hundreds of years.

The foundations of the debate go back at least to Aristotle, but it was the work of René Descartes and John Locke in the seventeenth century that set the stage for the most recent disputes about the existence of consciousness. In his quest to refute skepticism, Descartes found he could doubt the existence of everything in the universe (including his own body), but he could not doubt the fact that he was doubting (*Discourse on the Method*). Since doubt was a form of thought, the beginning of all knowledge for Descartes was in his consciousness that he was thinking: "*cogito ergo sum.*" Further, as noted in the last chapter, Descartes held that the body and the mind (soul) had separate existences: the former as a physical substance, *res extensa*; the latter as a spiritual one, *res cogitans*. The *res cogitans*—the "thing which thinks"—was considered an entity, with properties or faculties of its own.

The relationship between mind, consciousness, and personal identity was also examined by Locke in *An Essay concerning Human Understanding*. There he defined consciousness as "the perception of what passes in a man's own mind,"[1] and held that to find wherein personal identity consists, we must consider what *person* stands for;—which, I think, is a thinking intelligent being, that has reason and reflection, and can consider itself as itself, the same thinking thing, in different times and places; which it does only by that consciousness which is inseparable from thinking, and, as it seems to me, essential to it: it being impossible for any one to perceive without *perceiving* that he does perceive. When we see, hear, smell, taste, feel, meditate, or will anything, we know that we do so. Thus it is always as to our present sensations and perceptions: and by this every one is to himself that which he calls *self*. (Pp. 448–49)

This empirical perspective on consciousness and the self was continued in the eighteenth-century philosophy of David Hume. But Hume doubted the existence of a continuous *self*, of an immaterial entity that generates our consciousness:

For my part, when I enter most intimately into what I call *myself*, I always stumble on some particular perception or other, of heat or cold, light or shade, love or hatred, pain or pleasure. I never can catch *myself* at any time without a perception, and never can observe anything but the perception. When my perceptions are remov'd for any time, as by sound sleep; so long am I insensible of *myself*, and may truly be said not to exist. . . .

The mind is a kind of theatre, where several perceptions successively make their appearance; pass, re-pass, glide away, and mingle in an infinite variety of postures and situations. . . . The comparison of the theatre must not mislead us. They are the successive perceptions only, that constitute the mind; nor have we the most distant notion of the place, where these scenes are represented, or of the materials, of which it is compos'd.[2]

Hume thus echoed George Berkeley's maxim: *"esse est percipi"*— "to be is to be perceived." But, as David Ballin Klein observed, Hume "did not infer an independent percipient. Unlike Descartes, he was not saying 'perception is taking place, therefore I am a separate mind or soul or spirit. ' "[3]

This doubt of an immaterial thinker, of a *res cogitans*, became outright rejection in the psychology of William James. Although his views on consciousness changed over the years, James always held that it was not an entity, but rather a stream of thoughts.[4] He emphasized mental functions such as reasoning and remembering, rather than mental faculties such as "Reason" and "Memory." That James meant to repudiate the Cartesian perspective is clear from the following passage:

I believe that "consciousness" . . . is on the point of disappearing altogether. It is the name of a nonentity, and has no right to a place among first principles. Those who still cling to it are clinging to a mere echo, the faint rumor left behind by the disappearing "soul" upon the air of philosophy. . . .

To deny plumply that "consciousness" exists seems so absurd on the face of it—for undeniably "thoughts" do exist—that I fear some readers will follow me no farther. Let me then immediately explain that I mean only to deny that the word stands for an entity, but to insist most emphatically that it does stand for a function. There is, I mean, no aboriginal stuff or quality of being, contrasted with that of which material objects are made . . . but there is a function in experience which thoughts perform. . . . That function is *knowing*.[5]

But must we accept the existence of thoughts? John Watson, the founder of behaviorism, did not think so:

Behaviorism . . . leaves out speculations. You'll find in it no references to the intangibles—the unknown and the unknowable "psychic entities." The behaviorist has nothing to say of "consciousness." How can he? Behaviorism is a natural science. He has neither seen, smelled nor tasted consciousness nor found it taking part in any human reactions. How can he talk about it until he finds it in his path? His way—his method is to build a psychology without it. He does the same with the subdivisions of consciousness—such as sensations—perceptions—affections—will and the like. In behaviorism you find none of these grand old speculative bugaboos about which so many millions of pages have been so fruitlessly written.[6]

Almost 50 years later, B. F. Skinner took behaviorism back somewhat from this lofty position: "Methodological behaviorism and certain versions of logical positivism could be said to ignore consciousness, feelings, and states of mind, but radical behaviorism does not thus 'behead the organism.' "[7] Skinner offered two meanings of "consciousness": in the first, a person is said to be conscious if he is aware of stimuli arising from within his body; in the second, he is conscious when his "verbal community arranges contingencies under which he not only sees an object but sees that he is seeing it" (p. 220). In this latter sense, consciousness is a social product, and the types of experiences said to constitute consciousness will vary from one "verbal community" to another. But, Skinner concluded, the old-fashioned concept of consciousness was still of doubtful value:

Must we conclude that all those who have speculated about consciousness as a form of self-knowledge—from the Greeks to the British empiri-
cists to the phenomenologists—have wasted their time? Perhaps we
must. They deserve credit for directing attention to the relation between
a person and his environment . . . but they have directed inquiry away
from antecedent events in his environmental history. (P. 221)

For a half-century after Watson, American psychology was
dominated by behaviorism, and "the use of the term [consciousness]
was not allowed."[8] But over the last 20 years the study of consciousness has again come to center stage. It is not that behaviorism
has disappeared, but rather that cognitive and motivational factors
are so important in the lives of human beings that they could no
longer be overlooked. The phenomenal world is a conscious world,
even for behaviorists.

While psychologists debated the existence of consciousness, physicians continued to regard it as a useful concept. A patient's "level"
of consciousness, for example, has long been recognized as an important marker of his health. It is a bad prognostic sign if the patient's illness is characterized by a deterioration in consciousness
from alertness through drowsiness to stupor and coma. As well, certain forms of epilepsy (e.g., *petit mal* attacks) are clinically manifest
only by alterations in consciousness.

But the interest of physicians in the concept of consciousness
extends beyond the phenomenon as a dimension of alertness. Psychiatric patients complaining of *depersonalization*, for example, describe a pathological consciouness of self. They are awake and alert
but estranged or disconnected from themselves in some vital way.
They feel as if they are made of plastic or wood, and though they
know they are causing their limbs to move, they nonetheless claim
to feel like robots. As Jaspers observed: "The remarkable thing
about this particular phenomenon is that the individual, though he
exists, is no longer able to feel he exists. Descartes' 'cogito ergo sum'
(I think therefore I am) may still be superficially cogitated but it
is no longer a valid experience."[9]

CONSCIOUS DEFINED

Consciousness may be easier to defend than to define, a state
of affairs that seems to have changed little since 1904, when Ralph
Barton Perry observed:

There is no philosophical term at once so popular and so devoid of
standard meaning. How can a term mean anything when it is employed

to connote anything and everything, including its own negation? One hears of the object of consciousness and the subject of consciousness, and the union of the two in self-consciousness; of the private consciousness, the social consciousness, and the transcendental consciousness; the inner and the outer, the higher and the lower, the temporal and the eternal consciousness; the activity and the state of consciousness. Then there is consciousness-stuff, and unconscious consciousness, called respectively mind-stuff for short, and unconscious psychical states or subconsciousness to avoid a verbal contradiction. This list is not complete, but sufficiently amazing.[10]

The reason we have so much difficulty agreeing on a definition of *conscious* is that the term represents a disjunctive category. Disjunctive categories are those in which the basic concept behind the category can be embodied in several different ways.[11] A *citizen*, for example, "belongs" somewhere. Thus, someone can be a citizen of a country if he is born there, or if he lives there for a stipulated period, or if he marries a native. The *or* illustrates the point that the criteria for citizenship are equivalent.

The basic concept behind the category *consciousness* can be seen in its etymology. It is derived from the Latin *conscius*, whose roots are *com* (with) and *scire* (to know). But the "knowing," the awareness, at the center of consciousness can be satisfied if one is perceiving, or remembering, or willing, or even dreaming. Consciousness is not a single, indivisible thing, but rather a concept that can be exemplified and studied in various ways. And if we still cannot agree on how to define consciousness once and for all, we can at least measure its manifestations, both as the correlates of brain activities on which it depends, and from the reports of individuals who reflect upon their phenomenal worlds.

IN DEFENSE OF UNCONSCIOUS

Why is the term *unconscious* a negation of *conscious*? The reason for its derivative status may be that the concept of consciousness, with its links to the self, took precedence in the development of European thought:

The seventeenth century was the first period when the individual's experience of "consciousness" and "self-consciousness" was isolated and treated as a primary concept or value, the first principle of universal philosophies. . . .
In English "conscious" as meaning "inwardly sensible or aware" appears first in 1620, "consciousness" or "the state of being conscious" in

1678, and "self-consciousness" or "conscious of one's own thoughts, etc." in 1690.[12]

As Descartes had shown, rational awareness was the way in which the self and the universe were to be explained. The Cartesian emphasis on self-consciousness as the foundation of all knowledge cast doubt on the existence of mental processes of which the individual was not aware. Indeed, for Locke, the very idea of *unconscious thought* was impossible:

[A man] cannot *think* at any time, waking or sleeping, without being sensible of it. Our being sensible of it is not necessary to anything but to our thoughts; and to them it is; and to them it always will be necessary, till we can think without being conscious of it.[13]

And yet, despite this exaltation of consciousness, it was difficult to ignore the existence of unconscious processes. It had long been recognized that daydreaming and sleep were states of diminished self-awareness in which thinking of a kind occurred, and that vital functions of the body such as breathing took place without conscious control. But it was also apparent that some human actions were not "rational," that they could not be accounted for by events in the phenomenal world, and thus there came to be a growing sense of *unconscious* in another guise: as hidden mental processes that could shape conscious thought and behavior. The "discovery" of the unconscious in this latter sense was *"an unavoidable inference from experience,"*[14] and it began to be affirmed even as consciousness started its reign. Thus, in 1690, five months after the publication of Locke's *Essay*, a sometime friend of its author admonished him that "there may be Impressions made on the Mind, whereof we are not conscious, or which we do not perceive."[15]

For the next 200 years, many philosophers and physicians championed the existence of unconscious mental processes, and some even claimed that those processes, rather than conscious ones, were the foundation of human mental life. In 1704, for example, G. W. Liebniz also took issue with Locke's claims:

There are countless indications which lead us to think that there is at every moment an infinity of *perceptions* within us, but without apperception and without reflexion; that is to say, changes in the soul itself of which we are not conscious, because the impressions are either too small and too numerous or too closely combined, so that each is not distinctive enough by itself, but nevertheless in combination with others each has its effect and makes itself felt, at least confusedly, in the whole. . . .

In a word, *unconscious perceptions* are of as great use in pneumatics [the philosophy of mind] as imperceptible corpuscles are in physics; and it is as unreasonable to reject the one as the other on the ground that they are beyond the reach of our senses.[16]

But unconscious mental processes eventually came to be seen as more than mere building blocks of consciousness. They could be considered dynamic, as well as static, phenomena—as processes that initiated and influenced conscious mental life. Thus, Sir William Hamilton asked:

Are there, in ordinary, mental modifications,—*i.e.* mental activities and passivities, of which we are unconscious, but which manifest their existence by effects of which we are conscious? . . . In the question proposed, I am not only strongly inclined to the affirmative,—nay, I do not hesitate to maintain, that what we are conscious of is constructed out of what we are not conscious of,—that our whole knowledge, in fact, is made up of the unknown and the incognisable. . . . The sphere of our conscious modifications is only a small circle in the centre of a far wider sphere of action and passion, of which we are only conscious through its effects.[17]

By the last half of the nineteenth century, what had started as a faint counterpoint to the dominant theme of consciousness became a movement of its own. Though unconscious mental processes were still mysterious (hypnosis, after all, has yet to be explained), the leading physicians, psychologists, and philosophers of the day had accepted their existence and importance—so much so that in the decade following the publication of Eduard von Hartmann's *Philosophy of the Unconscious* in 1868, five other books appeared with the term *unconscious* in their titles.[18] From there, interest in and knowledge about unconscious processes has continued to grow, both in the laboratory and in the clinic. An example of recent experimental work on unconscious phenomena can be found in the studies of Benjamin Libet, a neurophysiologist.

Libet and his colleagues have investigated the readiness potential, a negative shift in the electrical activity of the brain that preceeds voluntary motor activity and can be recorded from the scalp. In a series of inventive experiments they found that,

since onset of [the readiness potential] regularly begins at least several hundreds of milliseconds before the appearance of a reportable time for awareness of any subjective intention or wish to act, it would appear that some neuronal activity associated with the eventual performance of the act has started well before any (recallable) conscious initiation or intervention could be possible. Put another way, the brain evidently "decides" to initiate or, at the least, prepare to initiate the act at a time before there is any reportable subjective awareness that such a decision has taken place. It is concluded that cerebral initiation even of a spontaneous voluntary act, of the kind studied here, can and usually does begin *unconsciously*.[19]

It is of interest that much experimental work on unconscious mental phenomena has been done by American psychologists, who had for so long tended to ignore the role of cognitive factors in behavior. As Howard Shevrin and Scott Dickman conclude in their review of such research, the "clear message from much recent thinking in psychology appears to be that behavior cannot be understood without taking conscious experience into account and that conscious experience cannot be fully understood without taking unconscious psychological processes into account."[20]

With so much support from psychology, physiology, philosophy, and psychiatry (not to mention its importance as the wellspring of creativity for artistic and intellectual movements such as Romanticism and Surrealism), it may be difficult to understand why the concept of an unconscious realm—"the" unconscious—has been so fiercely resisted by some of those most interested in mental life. In part, professional antagonism to "the" unconscious has arisen on theoretical grounds. James, for example, held that it was "the sovereign means for believing what one likes in psychology, and of turning what might become a science into a tumbling-ground for whimsies,"[21] while Watson, in a chapter entitled "The Myth of the Unconscious," referred to it as an outdated concept whose referents would better be described as "unverbalized behavior."[22]

But arguments against "the" unconscious have come from critics outside the scientific community as well as from within it, and a theme common to both groups has been their belief in the value of rational thought. According to Lancelot Law Whyte, many such critics have

tended to regard the unconscious as the realm of irrational forces threatening the social and intellectual order which the rational consciousness, they imagined, had built up over generations. Day was challenged by Night, the enlightenment of reason by the tempests and conflicts of intuition and instinct, the soul of man by a dark and frightening, but desperately attractive, inner spirit of temptation and surrender.[23]

This uneasiness about the unconscious came to cluster primarily around the theories of Freud. The reason for this cannot be only that Freud linked the unconscious with sexuality and other instinctual drives, for earlier writers had also done so. And it cannot be only because Freud's ideas represented a systematic account of unconscious mental life; other theorists had made similar attempts. Nor can it be simply that Freud's insights challenged the received opinions of his medical colleagues and found champions among the intellectual radicals of the day. Though all of these factors, and more, contribute to a distrust of the unconscious realm Freud described, a major reason must be found in his proposal that *all* mental life—normal as well as pathological—rested on particular sorts of unconscious forces. These forces were both primitive and powerful and came to constitute a kind of self-within-the-self that determined conscious thoughts and behaviors. Such ideas draw not only the contempt of those who scorn mental entities of any kind (conscious or unconscious) but also the ire of those who see that the highest purposes and creations of human culture are more than the disguised manifestations of simple or ignoble drives.

Though many characterizations of the unconscious have been offered (for it, like consciousness, is a disjunctive category), Freud's has anchored one end of the conscious-unconscious polarity in the minds of most psychiatrists. Though we can only treat of it briefly, it is to his definition that we now turn.

UNCONSCIOUS DEFINED

In "A Note on the Unconscious in Psycho-analysis," Freud presented his first detailed account of unconscious mental processes:

A conception . . . which is now *present* to my consciousness may become *absent* the next moment, and may become *present again*, after an interval, unchanged, and, as we say, from memory, not as a result of a fresh perception by our senses. It is this fact which we are accustomed to account for by the supposition that during the interval the conception has been present in our mind, although *latent* in consciousness. . . .

Now let us call "conscious" the conception which is present to our consciousness and of which we are aware. . . . As for latent conceptions . . . let them be denoted by the term "unconscious."

Thus an unconscious conception is one of which we are not aware, but the existence of which we are nevertheless ready to admit on account of other proofs or signs.[24]

One such "proof" could be found in posthypnotic suggestion, which led Freud from a purely descriptive view of the unconscious to a dynamic one. A subject who had been hypnotized to perform a certain action did so as soon as the thought of the action entered his awareness. Yet the real stimulus to the action had been the physician's order to the subject under hypnosis, and that order "did not reveal itself to consciousness, as did its outcome . . . it remained unconscious, and so it was *active and unconscious* at the same time" (p. 261).

Such active unconscious ideas were believed by Freud not only to characterize hypnosis but also to be at the root of hysterical and other neurotic symptoms, which represented the manifest effects of repressed unconscious ideas:

The term *unconscious*, which was used in the purely descriptive sense before, now comes to imply something more. It designates not only latent ideas in general, but especially ideas with a certain dynamic character, ideas keeping apart from consciousness in spite of their intensity and activity. . . .

The unconscious idea is excluded from consciousness by living forces which oppose themselves to its reception, while they do not object to other ideas. . . . Psycho-analysis leaves no room for doubt that the [fending off of] unconscious ideas is only provoked by the tendencies embodied in their contents. The next and most probable theory which can be formulated at this stage of our knowledge is the following. Unconsciousness is a regular and inevitable phase in the processes constituting our psychical activity; every psychical act begins as an unconscious one, and it may either remain so or go on developing into consciousness, according as it meets with resistance or not. (Pp. 262, 264)

Although this "topographical" model of mental functioning (which classified phenomena as unconscious, preconscious, and conscious) was eventually joined to a "structural" one (in which the mental apparatus was composed of id, ego, and superego), Freud continued to affirm the fundamental importance of a dynamic unconscious whose contents were subject to repression. Thinking in these terms brought a fresh and optimistic approach to the treatment of patients, such as those with hysterical disorders, whose complaints had previously been regarded by many as evidence of inherited degeneration or misbehavior. For Freud, the symptoms of these patients were to be understood as the disguised manifestations of repressed wishes, wishes whose content was usually sexual in nature. From his earliest work with hysterics, Freud was

anxious to show that sexuality does not simply intervene, like a *deus ex machina*, on one single occasion, at some point in the working of the processes which characterize hysteria, but that it provides the motive power for every single symptom, and for every single manifestation of a symptom. The symptoms of the disease are nothing else than *the patient's sexual activity*. . . . I can only repeat over and over again—for I never find it otherwise—that sexuality is the key to the problem of the psychoneuroses and of the neuroses in general. . . . I still await news of the investigations which are to make it possible to contradict this theorem or to limit its scope. What I have hitherto heard against it have been expressions of personal dislike or disbelief.[25]

It may have been that some of the "dislike or disbelief" of Freud's views were reactions to his claim that what characterized the unconscious life of disturbed patients also characterized the unconscious life of healthy people. Even such minor phenomena as slips of the tongue, habitual gestures, and the humming of tunes

are not so insignificant as people, by a sort of conspiracy of silence, are ready to suppose. They always have a meaning. . . . And it turns out that once again they give expression to impulses and intentions which have to be kept back and hidden from one's own consciousness, or that they are actually derived from the same repressed wishful impulses and complexes which we have already come to know as the creators of symptoms and the constructors of dreams. They therefore deserve to be rated as symptoms. . . . A man's most intimate secrets are as a rule betrayed by their help. . . .

As you already see, psycho-analysts are marked by a particularly strict belief in the determination of mental life. For them there is nothing trivial, nothing arbitrary or haphazard.[26]

Thus, for Freud, nothing was to be taken at face value, and, as can be seen from the following passage, the claims of an individual to have made a simple error might count for little against the authority of psychoanalytic theory:

In order to explain a slip of the tongue, for instance, we find ourselves obliged to assume that the intention to make a particular remark was present in the subject. We infer it with certainty from the interference with his remark which has occurred; but the intention did not put itself through and was thus unconscious. If, when we subsequently put it before the speaker, he recognizes it as one familiar to him, then it was only temporarily unconscious to him; but if he repudiates it as something foreign to him, then it was permanently unconscious.[27]

(Students of English history will recognize in this last sentence an example of Morton's Fork. John Morton, advisor to Henry VII, was responsible for a program of tax collection in which the rich were told they could obviously afford to contribute, while the poor were accused of having hidden their wealth.)

But repressed unconscious impulses were seen not only to determine the thoughts and behaviors of ordinary people; they were also believed to hold the key to an understanding of the greatest creations of the human spirit. Thus, though Freud reminded his readers that he was far from certain in his conclusion that the art of Leonardo da Vinci was a sublimated expression of repressed sexual impulses, he was still confident enough in his views to claim, "We must be content to emphasize the fact—which it is hardly any longer possible to doubt—that what an artist creates provides at the same time an outlet for his sexual desire."[28]

Freud's concept of the unconscious was a source of illumination and inspiration both within and outside the psychiatric community. And though the psychoanalytic movement he began eventually emphasized ego more than id and adaptation more than defense, and though motivations other than sexual ones were implicated in hysterical phenomena, Freud's claim for the importance of unconscious mental processes has never been abandoned.

As well as approbation, of course, there has been skepticism and repudiation. Thus, Alfred Adler and C. G. Jung disagreed with Freud as to the nature of basic unconscious motivations, and Watson and Popper found his views to be unscientific. But some of the most telling criticism was made by Jaspers, who nonetheless agreed with Freud on certain fundamental assumptions:

Psychic life . . . cannot be fully understood in terms of consciousness, nor is it to be grasped by consciousness alone. . . . Direct, accessible psychic experiences are like the foam on the sea's surface. The depths are inaccessible and can only be explored in an indirect and theoretical way. . . . In order to explain psychic life we have to work with extra-conscious mechanisms and unconscious events, which of course can never be visualised as such but can only be conceived in simile and symbol, whether physical or psychic.[29]

Jaspers reserved the term *unconscious* for psychic events that have actually been experienced by the individual but have gone unregarded or been forgotten. Such phenomena may be brought into consciousness under appropriate circumstances, including the techniques of psychoanalysis. "Extra-conscious" events, on the other hand, have never actually been experienced. They are processes in the brain, such as the discharge of neurons, whose existence may be inferred from their effects in the phenomenal world. For Jaspers, unconscious events are related to conscious ones through *under-standing* (Verstehen), while extraconscious events can be linked to conscious ones only through *explanation* (Erklären). Jaspers believed that Freud's failure to appreciate the distinction between understanding and explanation in the unconscious realm was a capital error.

Although Jaspers acknowledged Freud's meaningful insights into human behavior, he held that the "falseness of the Freudian claim lies in the mistaking of meaningful connections for causal connections. The claim is that *everything* in the psychic life, every psychic event, is *meaningful* (comprehensibly determined)" (p. 539). Jaspers, on the other hand, believed that the genesis of many psychic events in both normal and abnormal individuals was to be found in extraconscious processes, in brain mechanisms that could not be understood but only explained. Freud's claim to have developed a general theory of human mental life based on the understanding of particular meaningful connections in the lives of a few patients was therefore unjustified.

Despite such criticisms of his method, Freud maintained that psychoanalysis was a science and that the unconscious processes he described were akin to the fundamental mechanisms of the physical universe:

The hypothesis we have adopted of a psychical apparatus extended in space, expediently put together, developed by the exigencies of life, which gives rise to the phenomena of consciousness only at one particular point and under certain conditions—this hypothesis has put us in a position to establish psychology on foundations similar to those of any other science, such, for instance, as physics.[30]

From this perspective, the phenomenal world is not only determined by unconscious processes, but determined in a way that is inherently mechanical, as the vector sum of contending forces in the id, the ego, and the superego. Freud thought he had found the machine in the ghost of consciousness.

It is important to realize, however, that the unconscious mechanisms described by Freud are different from those in clocks or engines. The id, the ego, and the superego are not merely interconnected parts, assembled at a given time and functioning more or less smoothly to generate behavior. Rather, they compose a kind of mechanical or cybernetic self, powered by the instinctual drives and programmed to satisfy them as best it can. Exactly how the drives are satisfied varies from person to person, depending on constitutional factors and developmental experiences, but in every individual the mechanisms are the same. This unconscious self, with its own premises, intentions, and rules of conduct, is the hidden determinant of the phenomenal world, and it remains obscured from the conscious self unless revealed by the psychoanalyst.

The power of Freud's concept rests partly on its resemblance to the mechanisms of Newtonian physics and Darwinian biology, and in that resemblance lies its challenge to other views of human nature. If conscious mental life is devoid of accident, it is also devoid of freedom and, ultimately, of values—at least of values in the noblest sense of the word. For Freud, philosophy and religion were illusions derived from infantile needs,[31] and Hamlet's ambivalence was merely a riddle to be solved by reference to the Oedipus complex.[32] Our heroes and heroines are gone, and with them the meaning of many human aspirations.

## Thinking in Terms of Psychiatric Methodology

When psychiatrists speak of unconscious motivations and conflicts, they may only be revealing their ignorance of how the brain processes internal and external stimuli to generate behavior, the phenomenal world, and the sense of self. Freud believed this to be the case and throughout his career was prevented by the mind-brain disjunction from developing the kind of psychology he had originally thought possible. In 1895 Freud announced a bold project: "The intention is to furnish a psychology that shall be a natural science: that is, to represent psychical processes as quantitatively determinate states of specifiable material particles, thus making those processes perspicuous and free from contradiction."[33] Like those before and after him, however, Freud could not unite mind and brain, and in 1938, near the end of his career, he wrote:

We know two kinds of things about what we call our psyche (or mental life): firstly, its bodily organ and scene of action, the brain (or nervous system) and, on the other hand, our acts of consciousness, which are immediate data and cannot be further explained by any sort of description. Everything that lies between is unknown to us, and the data do not include any direct relation between these two terminal points of our knowledge.[34]

Since he could not derive individual mental states from discrete cerebral events, since his knowledge of the brain was inadequate to account for the symptoms of his patients, Freud proposed something to bridge the gap: a theory of the unconscious that seemed, in Jaspers's terms, to make understandable what could not be explained. The unconscious domain Freud depicted was inferred from his clinical observations, but it also reflected his views on the human condition. Those views are Freud's philosophy of life, not laws of Nature, and though they command respect, they do not compel assent.

REFLECTIONS ON THE FREUDIAN UNCONSCIOUS

Once Freud's approach to the unconscious is seen to rest on the method of understanding rather than on the method of explanation, its place in psychiatry as a means of interpretation can be better appreciated. We do not refer here to his specific theories about the composition, characteristics, or development of an unconscious self, for those are controversial matters even within psychoanalysis, but instead to his general idea that human behavior can be shaped by motivations and conflicts of which the conscious self is not aware. These hidden motivations and conflicts are proposed in order to make sense of thoughts, moods, and acts that would otherwise be mysterious. If used within the limits of the method of understanding, they enable a clinician to account for certain gaps in the patient's phenomenal world and to tell a life story that is coherent, dynamic, and meaningful.

In the case of Mr. B., for example, the proposal of an unconscious conflict over the expression of angry feelings both illuminates his illness and guides his treatment. It provides a meaningful theme that draws together important aspects of his personality, childhood experiences, and current situation, and it reveals a function for his pseudoseizures that makes sense of their occurrence. We come to understand Mr. B.'s spells as part of his life story rather than vainly trying to explain them as signs of his brain's dysfunction.

Jaspers saw the value of understanding hysterical phenomena in terms of unconscious processes, though he also warned of the dangers associated with this approach:

In all these understandable phenomena we have tried to see the *specific somatic content as psychically meaningful*; we have tried to see the somatic event as an essential in the psychic and social context of the individual. In this the respective relationship between body and psyche has remained unconscious yet in principle open to consciousness; if the patient gains understanding of the connection, this reverts back with healing effect on the somatic phenomena, always provided there is a change in the psychic attitude along with the mere intellectual understanding. And here we have reached the field of interpretation which is most seductive but dangerous to enter. There is no doubt that fundamental knowledge may be gained here, but nowhere else do genuine evidence and gross deception go so closely together. A wealth of possible experience seems to offer itself but with it come confusing ambivalences and mistaken acceptances of the first interpretation that comes to hand.[35]

Here Jaspers is reminding us that meaningful connections have certain properties and that these properties must be borne in mind if we wish to account for conscious thoughts and behaviors in terms of unconscious motivations and conflicts. "Confusing ambivalences" can arise, for example, from the fact that many different (and even opposite) meaningful connections can be proposed for the same event, so that it is sometimes difficult to decide which of them is the most appropriate one to employ. As well, we can mistakenly accept "the first interpretation that comes to hand" because the self-evident quality of meaningful connections can generate a powerful sense of conviction, even when empirical support for the interpretation is minimal. This is a special danger when unconscious mechanisms are suggested, for it is with such mechanisms that the tendency of meaningful connections to follow the "hermeneutic round" is most clearly seen.

Given a theoretical preconception about the type of unconscious motivation that is symbolically expressed in a certain disorder, for example, it is quite easy to interpret the patient's experience in terms of that symbolism. This hermeneutic reading of the patient's life story then serves to reinforce our opinion that the unconscious motivation is actually present, though manifest in a disguised form. The ease with which conscious events and unconscious processes can be linked by meaningful theories makes such theories "most seductive," for they promise to simplify that which is complicated and to illuminate that which is mysterious. Indeed, those who hold that conscious thoughts and behaviors are determined by unconscious motivations and conflicts lay claim to a special kind of knowledge: knowledge that is elusive, yet ultimate; knowledge that is potentially open to everyone, but in practice possessed by few; knowledge that is derived, not from the hypothetico-deductive methods of the natural sciences but from the interpretative methods of the humanities.

Unconscious mechanisms of the type Freud proposed thus give

meaning to life stories that would otherwise be incoherent and in-complete. They confer intentionality on acts that seem without pur-pose, and they link even the most bizarre and self-destructive be-havior to aspirations and predicaments that can be articulated in human terms. As such meaningful connections are made, order re-places chaos and rational understanding becomes possible.

It is important to note here that meaningful connections based on unconscious mechanisms not only restore order; they impose it. Freud's decision to rest such connections on the instinctual drives made it possible to account for the occurrence and persistence of thoughts and acts that seemed inexplicable or repugnant, since, in his view, the instinctual drives were so compelling that, sooner or later, in one form or another, their effects would be felt and behav-iors determined.

The recognition of disguised drives is, as noted above, part of the hermeneutic process that operates whenever unconscious mech-anisms are thought responsible for events in the phenomenal world. If such drives are "discovered" to be the "real" motivations behind actions and choices, it follows that the conscious self is only the most superficial aspect of the "true" self, whose dark, primitive core must be exposed by psychoanalytic techniques if human nature is to be fully understood.

In the end, the knowledge claimed by those who invoke an un-conscious realm of motivations and conflicts is gnostic in character, for it is held to be essential to the salvation of both individuals and mankind. Freud himself saw such a role for the theory he had de-veloped:

We do not consider it at all desirable for psycho-analysis to be swallowed up by medicine and to find its last resting-place in a text-book of psy-chiatry under the heading "Methods of Treatment." . . . It deserves a better fate and, it may be hoped, will meet with one. As a "depth-psychology," a theory of the mental unconscious, it can become indispen-sable to all the sciences which are concerned with the evolution of hu-man civilization and its major institutions such as art, religion and the social order. . . . The use of analysis for the treatment of the neuroses is only one of its applications; the future will perhaps show that it is not the most important one. . . . Our civilization imposes an almost intolera-ble pressure on us and it calls for a corrective. Is it too fantastic to ex-pect that psycho-analysis in spite of its difficulties may be destined to the task of preparing mankind for such a corrective? Perhaps once more an American may hit on the idea of spending a little money to get the "social workers" of his country trained analytically and to turn them into a band of helpers for combating the neuroses of civilization.

"Aha! a new kind of Salvation Army!"

Why not? Our imagination always follows patterns.[36]

Freud proposed an encompassing theory of human nature, and though it began with Anna O. and Dora, it soon extended to Hamlet and Prometheus—from the disorders of the individual to the disorders of the civilization. In Freud's work, the discourse is one of meaning rather than science, of myths rather than molecules. His claims about the unconscious self and its mechanisms have made a powerful impression within psychiatry and beyond it, but we must remember that they are claims, not proofs. As Freud's thought moved inevitably from the world of the clinic to the world at large, it revealed both the scope and the limitations of *Verstehen*.

"CONSCIOUS," "UNCONSCIOUS," AND THE PRACTICE
OF PSYCHIATRY

A major problem with the terms *conscious* and *unconscious* is that they are often treated as if they could be sharply demarcated from one another. Though sometimes we can be certain whether or not a patient is consciously producing his symptoms, at other times—as in the case of Mr. B.—the distinction is quite difficult.

This should not be surprising, given the complexity of human motivation. In the end, it often comes down to clinical judgment, and in doubtful cases that judgment should be reserved until we know the patient better. To assume, with hysterical phenomena, that conscious motivation always exists (and that patients are trying to decieve us) or that unconscious motivation always exists (and that patients are deceiving themselves) is to trivialize the problem.

But the cost of a doctrinaire position at one or the other extreme of the polarity of conscious and unconscious is more than that involved in the care of a particular patient or in the treatment of hysterical behaviors in general. Whether psychiatrists like it or not, the public often looks to them for opinions on important issues, such as the circumstances in which someone should or should not be held responsible for his actions. The implications of this polarity thus extend beyond the clinic to the courtroom and the statehouse.

Psychiatry's domain is the phenomenal world, and the phenomenal world is a conscious one. If all psychiatric disorders could be comprehended by reference to conscious processes (or to brain events), psychiatrists would have no need to postulate an unconscious realm of motivations and dispositions. As it is, however, there are gaps in the phenomenal world that can neither be explained in neurological terms nor immediately understood in meaningful ones. Under certain circumstances, then, psychiatrists propose and attempt to identify unconscious processes that give coherence to their formulations and direction to their treatments. In this way, the unconscious will be emphasized when we wish to remember that perceptions and decisions can occur without conscious awareness and that parts of the past, though seemingly forgotten, can be carried into the present to shape our thoughts and behaviors. Self-reflection will eventually reveal some of these things, but many of them lie beyond its power.

We will emphasize conscious processes, on the other hand, if we wish to develop treatments based on self-understanding and self-control and to protect our patients from the reductionism of meaningful connections that debase achievement as nothing but the disguised expression of some hidden impulse. Consciousness is the triumph of evolution, and its development has freed human beings from reflex responses to their external environments and internal drives. Indeed, to be fully human is to be a conscious, reflective, and deciding self.

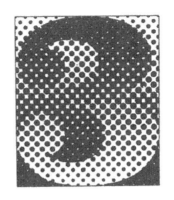

*Implications
of Ambiguity*

# 5

# Hebraic
# & Hellenic

Despite their many differences, materialist neuroscience, Freudian psychoanalysis, and Watsonian behaviorism are alike in seeking either to reduce the phenomenal world to something else or to eliminate it completely. For neuroscientists, the world of the self is an epiphenomenon of brain processes; for psychoanalysts, it represents the disguised derivatives of an unconscious realm; for behaviorists, it is a "speculative bugaboo," an unnecessary and obfuscating notion. Though in practice the phenomenal world is the point of contact between psychiatrists and their patients, each of these theoretical perspectives regards it as the manifestation of something else, something more basic and hence more important.

This reductionistic way of thinking about the phenomenal world influences not only the practice of psychiatry but also contemporary beliefs about human nature. In looking for the essence of that nature "beneath" the phenomenal world, there is a danger of trivializing the idea, and the value, of the conscious self.

For us, the essential qualities of human beings are to be found in the domain of personal consciousness, in the realm of the self. Though the phenomenal world is tied to the brain, though it emerges in part from unconscious processes, and though it is made manifest through behavior, the phenomenal world and the sense of self are what make human beings *human* beings. In this chapter, we will explore some of the consequences for psychiatric practice of this opinion, but before doing so, we must return briefly to the polarity of mind and brain to establish our argument.

### The Polarity of Mind and Brain Revisited

Mind and brain are separate realms of discourse. In the former, we speak of thoughts, moods, and conflicts; in the latter, of neurotransmitters, receptors, and enzymes. Mind and brain use different languages, and there is no Rosetta stone to translate the one into the other. If delusions could be explained by synaptic inhibition and broken promises by membrane potentials, then human beings would be machines and the self a matter of molecules.

As it is, selves and their phenomenal worlds are isolated from the brain. By "isolated" we do not mean they are independent of the central nervous system, but rather that talking in terms of selves is not the same thing as talking in terms of brains. From the viewpoint of the neuron, selves are invisible.

This fact is nowhere more evident than in the practice of psychiatry, where the complaints of many patients can be articulated and understood only in the idiom of selves. As Jaspers observed:

In physical illness we so resemble the animals [creatures whose destiny is determined by natural laws] that experiments on the latter can be used to reach an understanding of vital bodily function in humans, though the application may be neither simple or direct. But the concept of human psychic illness introduces a completely new dimension. Here the incompleteness and vulnerability of human beings and their freedom and infinite possibilities are themselves a cause of illness. In contrast with animals, man lacks an inborn, perfected pattern of adaptation. He has to acquire a way of life as he goes along. Man is not merely pattern, he patterns himself.[1]

The patterns human beings choose for themselves can fail for many reasons, ranging from immature judgments to bodily diseases. Whatever the cause of the failure, however, its effects are felt by a self, an individual whose life plan has now gone awry and who faces his "incompleteness and vulnerability" more than ever. Psychiatrists may be asked to help reformulate a life plan by such an injured self, and how they go about doing so will reflect not only their professional skills but also their views on human nature. The extent to which the patient is regarded as a subject/agent or an object/organism is not only a matter for differential diagnosis but also for what we see as a polarity of world views that is conceptualized in the terms *Hebraic* and *Hellenic*.

## The Polarity of Hebraic and Hellenic

MATTHEW ARNOLD

The terms *Hellenism* and *Hebraism* were used by Matthew Arnold in the late nineteenth century to indicate conflicting elements in the human spirit: Hellenism valued the intellectual side of human nature amd emphasized right thinking; Hebraism valued the moral side and emphasized right conduct. Though both had the same goal—the perfection of mankind—they pursued their aims in very different ways:

To get rid of one's ignorance, to see things as they are, and by seeing them as they are to see them in their beauty, is the simple and attractive ideal which Hellenism holds out before human nature. . . . Hellenism, and human life in the hands of Hellenism, is invested with a kind of aërial ease, clearness, and radiancy; they are full of what we call sweetness and light. Difficulties are kept out of view, and the beauty and rationalness of the ideal have all our thoughts. . . . But there is a saying which I have heard attributed to Mr. Carlyle about Socrates . . . which excellently marks the essential point in which Hebraism differs from Hellenism. "Socrates," this saying goes, "is terribly *at ease in Zion*." Hebraism . . . has always been severely preoccupied with an awful sense of the impossibility of being at ease in Zion; of the difficulties which oppose themselves to man's pursuit or attainment of that perfection of which Socrates talks so hopefully. . . . It is all very well to talk of getting rid of one's ignorance, of seeing things in their reality, seeing them in their beauty; but how is this to be done when there is something which thwarts and spoils all our efforts?

This something is *sin*. . . . Under the name of sin, the difficulties of knowing oneself and conquering oneself which impede man's passage to perfection, become, for Hebraism, a positive, active entity hostile to man . . . which it is the main business of our lives to hate and oppose.[2]

Arnold was interested in Hellenism and Hebraism as approaches to mankind's improvement and set his argument in terms of history and religion—perspectives somewhat removed from the person-to-person encounter that is the essence of psychiatric practice. For Arnold, the issue was a dialectic involving themes in the life of a culture; for psychiatrists, the issue is a dialogue involving meaning in the life of a self.

What does the patient make of his circumstances? Does he really want to change? How can he be helped to re-establish a life plan? These questions do not emerge directly from Arnold's treatment of Hebraism and Hellenism, but the polarity he proposed has been given a contemporary interpretation, and therein we find answers more directly related to the issue of psychiatry and the self.

WILLIAM BARRETT

Arnold, who wrote in a Victorian age scarred by doctrinaire conflict, proposed a view of human nature that championed synthesis rather than sectarianism: "Hebraism and Hellenism are, neither of them, the *law* of human development, as their admirers are prone to make them; they are, each of them, *contributions* to human development" (pp. 170–71). Arnold cautioned his readers about the dangers of unreflective confidence in their beliefs; William Barrett, writing in the mid-twentieth century, warned his audience about the dangers of not having any beliefs at all, of not having any faith, of not becoming *engaged* in their lives. For Barrett, the Greeks

were the first thinkers in history; they discovered the universal, the abstract and timeless essences, forms, and Ideas. The intoxication of this discovery (which marked nothing less than the earliest emergence and differentiation of the rational function) led Plato to hold that man lives only insofar as he lives in the eternal.

There follows for the Greek the ideal of *detachment* as the path of wisdom which only the philosopher can tred.[3]

If Plato and his eternal realm of essences represented Hellenism, then Job and his confrontation with God were emblematic of Hebraism:

The Hebrew . . . proceeds not by the way of reason but by the confrontation of the whole man, Job, in the fullness and violence of his passion with the unknowable and overwhelming God. And the final solution for Job lies not in the rational resolution of the problem, any more than it ever does in life, but in a change and conversion of the whole man. The relation between Job and God is a relation between an I and a Thou, to use Martin Buber's terms. Such a relation . . . is not the confrontation of two rational minds each demanding an explanation that will satisfy reason. The relation between Job and God is on the level of existence and not of reason. Rational doubt . . . never enters Job's mind, even in the very paroxysm of his revolt. His relation to God remains one of faith from start to finish. . . . Job says,"*Though he slay me, yet will I trust in him,*" but he adds what is usually not brought to our attention as emphatically as the first part of his saying: "*But I will maintain my own ways before him.*" Job retains his own identity ("his own ways") in confronting the Creator before whom he is as Nothing. (Pp. 73–74)

For Barrett, as an existentialist philosopher, modern civilization needs the Hebrew ideals of faith and commitment more than it does the Greek ideals of intellect and detachment. In using this Hebraic—Hellenic polarity, neither Barrett nor Arnold was making an oversimplified comparison between two very complex cultures. Rather, they saw in the Hebrew and Greek traditions a central tension in Western thought, a tension that we find most illuminating for the topic of psychiatry and the self.

Though the Hebraic—Hellenic polarity raises the contrast between doing and knowing, engagement and detachment, belief and skepticism, here we will emphasize how it leads us to consider what it means to be a self and how that meaning informs our practice. To discover the nature of selfhood (which is to say the nature of human beings), the Greeks and Hebrews might have asked very different questions: from the Hellenic perspective, "What is Man?"; from the Hebraic, "Who am I?"

HUMAN NATURE AND THE MEANING OF THE SELF

The difference between the Hellenic and Hebraic approaches has important implications for psychiatric practice, since it raises the issue of whether patients (and, indeed, all human beings) are best regarded as object/organisms or subject/agents. The Greeks, as exemplified by the pre-Socratic philosophers, tried to explain the natural world, to discern its forms and expose its workings. They were interested in the universal rather than the particular; in the abstract rather than the concrete; in classes rather than individuals. A characterization of human nature based on the Hellenic question, "What is Man?" might therefore contain two fundamental attributes.

First, human beings are animal beings. Our physical structures, experiential capacities, and developmental schedules are biologically determined rather than personally decided. Puberty, for example, simply *occurs*—we do not choose it and, under normal circumstances, we cannot avoid it. It is a fact of Nature. Puberty changes not only our appearance and behavior but also our phenomenal world and sense of self. Though we remain males or females, many of our interests, desires, and experiences are transformed from those of boys and girls to those of men and women.

But if biological determinism is usually evident through normal processes like those of puberty, it can also act through pathological mechanisms, such as those found in certain psychiatric disorders.

In conditions like Alzheimer's disease (where there is an established neuropathology) and manic-depressive illness (where a neuropathology is strongly suspected), the patient finds himself in the grip of something that distorts his phenomenal world and fragments his sense of self. He cannot reverse the process, though he desperately wishes to do so. Here human biology overrides human choice, and a pattern is imposed rather than embraced. If psychiatrists can reverse the pathological mechanism, if they can alter a fact of Nature, they can often restore the patient's phenomenal world, his sense of self, and his capacity for choice in the future.

The second characteristic to emerge from the Hellenic question, "What is Man?" is that human beings are cultural beings. Our phenomenal worlds and self-images are shaped by the roles and relationships that cultures provide. Though social forces may not be as inherently determining of experience and behavior as biological processes are, they can nonetheless influence patterns of life in a most powerful way. In some cultures, for instance, belonging to a family takes precedence over being an individual, and just as the family name is written before the personal name, so, too, family issues are thought about and dealt with before individual matters are.

Culture exerts its effects more through meanings and values than through science and technology. What is considered desirable or undesirable, good or bad, informs the choices and affects the health of individual citizens. The risk of becoming an alcoholic, for example, varies as a function of social policy: If the production and consumption of alcohol are promoted for economic reasons (e.g., to benefit distillers), the prevalence of alcohol abuse rises.[4]

From the perspective of Hellenism, human beings tend to be seen as special kinds of object/organisms whose behavior is determined and influenced by the forces of biology and culture. (Here neuroscience, psychoanalysis, and behaviorism agree.) From the perspective of Hebraism, however, with its focus on the particular rather than the universal, with its question, "Who am I?" rather than "What is Man?", individual human beings emerge from the background of the species as subject/agents who can choose to "maintain their own ways" in the face of biology, culture, and even God.

The ancient Hebrews fashioned a code of individual moral responsibility that is evident in Job's lament:

Let the Almighty state his case against me!

If my accuser had written out his indictment,
I would not keep silence and remain indoors.
No! I would flaunt it on my shoulder
and wear it like a crown on my head;
I would plead the whole record of my life
and present that in court as my defense.

Here is a conscious self who, having chosen a way of life, now struggles to understand the implications of his acts and the ultimate purpose of his existence. In our view, this conscious, reflective, deciding self is the locus of human nature, for it is in the domain of the self, in the phenomenal world, that values are weighed and choices are taken. We see this clearly in psychiatric practice, when patients confront pivotal questions: "Will you stop abusing drugs? . . . Can you understand your father's position? . . . How will you tell your children you have Huntington's disease?" Such questions are not asked of plastic neural systems, unconscious tripartite entities, or mindless organisms engaged in verbal behavior but of conscious selves who, despite the forces of biology and culture, and sometimes despite their own wishes, can and must choose one way of life rather than another.

## The Hebraic-Hellenic Polarity and the Practice of Psychotherapy

The issue of selves choosing to live one way rather than another is at the heart of psychotherapy, an endeavor in which the tension between Hebraic and Hellenic reasoning is clearly seen. At first glance, psychotherapy seems mostly a matter for the Hebraic perspective, since psychotherapists try to understand each patient as an individual; to enter his phenomenal world; to appreciate the complex and interrelated themes of his life story. But as psychiatrists gain experience in psychotherapy, as they stand back from the phenomenal worlds and life stories of particular patients, they begin to see that certain characteristics, intentions, and conflicts recur from patient to patient—not in exactly the same combinations, perhaps, but with enough consistency to form recognizable patterns.

Such patterns are not evident to beginners, and when they present a case to their teachers, they often recount every detail of the history and mental status examination, lest they do an injustice to the patient's individuality. Their teachers, on the other hand, are likely to summarize many of those details by saying, as in the case of Mr. B.: "He's an obsessional person and, like other obsessionals, he has difficulty in experiencing and expressing his emotions. Mr. B. is upset now because the future of his engagement and employment are uncertain and—again like other obsessionals—he finds uncertainty distressing."

In making such a formulation, the teacher proposes that the patient's complaint can be understood in terms of the neurotic paradigm, which identifies a relationship between potential, provocation, and response.[5] In the case of Mr. B., the potential is found in his obsessional traits, the provocation in his uncertain circumstances, and the response in his unexpressed anger and pseudoseizures. This formulation is useful in psychotherapy not only because it helps us to appreciate how the patient's distress may have developed, but also because it allows us to predict that distress will recur unless the patient can diminish his vulnerabilities or avoid situations that expose them.

And yet, by standing back from the patient in this Hellenic way, might there not be a tendency to overlook other aspects of his personality and circumstances, to stop listening to his unique life story, because his complaints have already been categorized as but one example of a more general phenomenon? If the abstraction comes to stand for the individual, the psychotherapist could miss those details that set this patient apart from others and that, if recognized, would demand alterations in the treatment plan. On the other hand, to ignore obvious similarities among patients and their responses to treatment might needlessly prolong both the course of psychotherapy and the patient's distress.

How can we balance this tension between individuals and types, particulars and abstractions, tailor-made interventions and standarized techniques? This manifestation of the Hebraic-Hellenic polarity is intrinsic to the practice of psychotherapy, but it is seen more by the psychotherapist than by the patient. For the patient, the Hellenic question, "What is Man?" has little interest; for him, the only meaningful question is the Hebraic one, "Who am *I*?"

"WHO AM I?"—A HELLENIC ANSWER

One answer to the patient's question is that, at present, he is likely to be a demoralized person. Jerome Frank sees demoralization as a feature common to the phenomenal worlds of many patients in psychotherapy:

They are conscious of having failed to meet their own expectations or those of others, or of being unable to cope with some pressing problem. They feel powerless to change the situation or themselves. In severe cases they fear that they cannot even control their own feelings.[6]

From the psychotherapist's point of view, then, the patient may be identified as a demoralized person, but it is often possible to depict him as a particular kind of demoralized person, as one with a certain pattern of personality traits. In the case of Mr. B., for example, Leon Salzman's description of obsessional traits and their consequences is apt:

The efforts at controlling his emotions may result in a paucity of emotional displays, but they cannot eliminate the enormous ground swells of feeling which are stored up. These untapped emotional sources may periodically burst out, either in minor ways . . . or in explosive major eruptions. . . . After awhile the accumulation may be great enough so that the expression of such feelings might be excessive even if the stimulus were minor.[7]

Although the issue of personality traits and their assessment is problematic, there is ample evidence to support the claim that at least some of them are valid concepts and that they render individuals vulnerable to distress in characteristic ways.[8]

To reason about patients in terms of potential, provocation, and response demonstrates the Hellenic approach to psychotherapy and, in the process, gives a general answer to the "Who am I?" question. This reasoning does not, however, necessarily imply that all patients have the same vulnerabilities or that they all face the same circumstances. A tendency to reach such conclusions is inherent in the Hellenic approach and sometimes leads to universal claims about patients in psychotherapy.

Universal claims can easily be recognized in pronouncements about the "essential cause" of neurotic symptoms and "the best" technique of psychotherapy. Such assertions are usually made by well-intentioned clinicians who mistake understanding for explanation, and whose enthusiasm and self-confidence can lead them to dismiss requests for objective evidence supporting their views as the petty criticism of doubters who refuse to see what is self-evident. These psychotherapists *believe*, they have *faith*, that their maxims are facts, and under the guise of answering the Hebraic question— "Who am I?"—they answer instead the Hellenic question—"What is Man?"—in a most Hebraic way.

"WHO AM I?"—A HEBRAIC ANSWER

In the end, psychotherapy is an individual matter. Although the patient may be appreciated as someone of a given personality type who reacts with characteristic symptoms to particular stresses, information of that sort never fully answers the question, "Who am *I*?"

The answer cannot be ready-made, in part because traits and symptoms and stresses are general in nature and do not substitute for a detailed knowledge of the patient's phenomenal world and life history. But more important, perhaps, is the fact that psychotherapy is not only a process of discovery; it is also a process of creation. The patient's sense of who he was and is (and will turn out to be) depends to some extent on how the psychotherapist tells his life story.

The procedure of telling a life story is not simply one of assembling all the facts and arranging them in chronological order.[9] Instead, the life story is a plausible and coherent *narrative* that reconstructs the present state of affairs. It starts at a certain time in the patient's life and draws together particular information about him into a linear perspective that makes his distress seem the logical, and sometimes even the inevitable, outcome of his past.

As a life story is told, then, certain things will be deemed essential and others trivial. In the case of Mr. B., for example, it may be more important to note that he was resentful of the attention paid his epileptic brother than it is to recall that he had a tonsillectomy at age five years. The theme of envy and disappointment in this story is given much more weight in understanding his current symptoms than the fact that he had minor surgery at a vulnerable age. It is this process of judging the eventual significance of events that makes the life story more than a chronicle.

Our ability to tell life stories in this way is based on our capacity to make meaningful connections. As we come to understand—in the sense of *Verstehen*—the relationship between event and emotion, intention and consequence, we come to appreciate the connectedness of things and begin to see them coalesce into an individual life story of increasing depth and complexity.

THE LIFE STORY'S AUTHOR

Although the patient provides most of the information on which his life story is based, the author of that story is the psychotherapist, for it is the latter who determines what will be used, what held in reserve, and what discarded. In this way, the psychotherapist "functions more as a pattern maker than a pattern finder."[10] Should he be theory-bound, for example, the psychotherapist will end up telling the same few stories over and over again, and much of the information contributed by the patient will be ignored in favor of a plot that has been used many times before. If this occurs, the psychotherapist has fallen into the Hellenic trap of thinking in terms of Platonic Ideas, of archtypal stories (such as the Oedipus complex), that may not do justice to the events of the patient's life.

Because no single collection of theory-based stories can approximate the variety and complexity of the human condition, it is wise for psychotherapists to familiarize themselves with at least several meaningful approaches that can be used as reference points in the telling of life stories. For one patient, a Freudian outline based on sexuality might serve; for another, Adler's views on inferiority would be apt; for a third, the Sullivanian emphasis on insecurity could be illuminating. Doctrinaire consistency may be confidence building, especially for beginners,[11] but it limits the vocabulary of psychotherapists and thus the range of stories they can tell. As Hilde Bruch observed:

Learning specific theories and therapeutic techniques, psychoanalytic or otherwise, may be stimulating and give the reassurance that one has been let in on some secret knowledge; to some it may be of help in organizing observations. But the beginner needs to realize that this knowledge does not give him any help when he sits down with a patient. It does not tell you what to say to a patient or what to listen for, and it may even make you focus on something which, according to the theory, should be there and thus stand in the way of hearing what the patient is trying to say.[12]

Unless we keep listening for what the patient is trying to say, the stories we tell will be taken more from books than from lives, and they will lack that sensitive understanding of an individual's distress that is essential to the psychotherapeutic relationship.

THE PSYCHOTHERAPEUTIC RELATIONSHIP

So far, psychotherapy has been discussed as if it rested solely on the telling of a life story, as if it were fundamentally a matter of exchanging information. While the importance of clarification, interpretation, and instruction cannot be denied, especially in counseling and in the briefer cognitive and behavioral therapies, such processes are not in themselves sufficient to help many patients face their "incompleteness and vulnerability" and change their life plans accordingly. If psychotherapy is a type of existential confrontation, patients need more than information to persevere.

As a life story is being told, as issues are being clarified and interpretations offered, the patient and the psychotherapist are drawn together into a relationship that sustains the patient in the midst of his distress and persuades him to hope. This relationship can itself be thought of in existential terms—as a kind of *I-Thou* encounter that is, in its own way, as lopsided as the one between Job, who reveals all, and God, who is unknowable—but however it is conceptualized, it is on the relationship established, rather than the information exchanged, that psychotherapy ultimately rests. It is probably this more than anything else that accounts for the effectiveness of so many different schools of psychotherapy; while each interprets distress in its own terms, all provide a relationship that combats demoralization, promotes insight, and encourages change.[13] Even lack of familiarity with the formal techniques of psychotherapy does not cancel the beneficial effects of this relationship, which is why inexperienced, though genuinely concerned and empathic, medical students can be successful as psychotherapists.[14]

The motivating power of psychotherapy depends more on Hebraic engagement than it does on Hellenic detachment. The patient is engaged to the extent that he suffers; the psychotherapist, to the extent that he cares. Caring, as Frank observes,

does not necessarily imply approval, but rather a determination to persist in trying to help no matter how desperate the patient's condition or how outrageous his behavior. Thus the therapeutic relationship always implies genuine acceptance of the sufferer, if not for what he is, then for what he can become.[15]

The patient and the psychotherapist must have faith that their work can succeed and that their trust in one another is warranted. Although knowledge, detachment, and other Hellenic virtues are important in the study and practice of psychotherapy, without engagement, psychotherapy loses its passion and, consequently, much of its power.

We use the word *passion* quite deliberately here, for the bond that develops between the patient and the psychotherapist is compounded of many emotions. It is the responsibility of the psychotherapist to insure that those emotions are used as a force for good in the patient's life. Sometimes he accomplishes this by making the nature of the emotion public (as when he identifies a "transference reaction" to the patient), while at other times he does it by remaining silent (as when he chooses not to show his frustration because he knows it will make the patient more demoralized). What to say now? What to do now? For the psychotherapist, definitive answers to these questions lie not in Hellenic theory, which can only guide practice in general ways, but in a detailed understanding of the patient's life story, in a commitment to his welfare, and in a Hebraic code of professional conduct and individual moral responsibility that recognizes the power of the psychotherapeutic relationship to do harm as well as good.

## Conclusion

We have used the Hebraic-Hellenic polarity to represent contrasting viewpoints on human nature and psychotherapy, but they are only two from among the many perspectives that are relevant to psychiatric practice. A multiplicity of viewpoints on human nature—scientific, economic, historical, philosophical, religious—have arisen because the phenomenal world and the sense of self can neither be constructed from the raw materials of the physical universe nor derived from a "unified field theory" that integrates all human qualities and potentials into a single, comprehensive system. As we find in the contrast between Hebraism and Hellenism, each viewpoint conceptualizes mankind in a distinct way.

Although this fact might lead some beginners in psychiatry to the sense that a choice among world views is merely a question of taste, it is our opinion that multiple viewpoints are essential and that, because each makes different assumptions and generates different consequences, the selection of one rather than another is a matter of great moment. Hebraism and Hellenism, for example, are complementary views of human nature in that each makes up for what the other lacks, but they are also fundamentally different in character and must be appreciated as such. Psychiatrists should therefore know when to be Hebrews and when to be Greeks.

The practice of psychiatry demands a body of knowledge and a set of values, and we must work as hard to acquire the one as the other. In the process of caring for patients, we think about ourselves, not only as physicians but also as individuals, since we are called upon to answer both Hellenic questions ("What are the genetics of manic-depressive disorder? . . . How do neuroleptic drugs work?") and Hebraic ones ("What do *I* consider normal behavior, appropriate aspirations, sufficient happiness? . . . Am *I* prepared to interfere with this person's liberty to preserve his life?")

In the following chapters we will explore the polarities of patient-client and autonomy-paternalism, two aspects of the physician-patient relationship that lead us to consider what we know *and* what we do. Though so far in the book our stance has been basically a descriptive and methodological one, as we discuss the implications of psychiatry's ambiguity for the conduct of its practitioners, we will become more prescriptive as well.

# 6
# Patient
# & Client

## The Professional Relationship

At rounds one day, a student nurse was asked to comment on the treatment plan that had been developed for one of our patients. She began by saying, "When I spoke with the client yesterday, he was very depressed," and throughout her remarks she continued to refer to the patient as "the client." When asked why she had done so, she said her instructors had taught her to use "client" because "it makes the patients more equal to us." The implication of her answer—that there is something inherently depreciatory in the term *patient*—led us to wonder why that venerable word should have acquired a pejorative connotation. If nurses were going to join many social workers and clinical psychologists in finding "patient" distasteful, what were we and our physician-colleagues missing, since none of us (so far as we knew) had ever used the word *client* to refer to those in our care?

It might be that calling patients *clients* would emphasize that we are in their service; that their needs, rather than ours, are primary. Or we might use the word *client* to remind ourselves that patients should, to the extent possible, be active participants in their treatment; that our job is usually to advise, not to decide. As well, perhaps calling patients *clients*, like calling mentally subnormal children *exceptional*, would lessen an unfortunate stigma and enable us to see more clearly the person behind the label.

Finally, the student nurse's use of *client* might be understood in light of a changing self-awareness among nurses. This interpretation receives some support from a textbook of psychiatric nursing whose glossary defines both *patient* and *client* as "a consumer of health services" but notes that the former is a "medical model" term, while the latter "is used instead of *patient* by some mental health professionals who oppose the medical model of mental disorder."[1] To the authors of that textbook, the "medical model" not only represents a certain perspective on the causes and treatments of psychiatric disorders but is also a way of organizing care in which the views of physicians predominate over those of patients and other professional members of the interdisciplinary team. They decry this practice and propose instead that team leadership should be flexible and that "the model for intervention and change" in patient care should be "one of negotiation and advocacy" (p. 6).

*Negotiation* and *advocacy* are words that seem more suited to lawyers and politicians than to physicians and nurses, and yet they are terms found increasingly in the discourse of medicine. Though the difference between *patient* and *client* may seem trivial, the issue it represents is symptomatic of fundamental changes in medical practice, including the physician-patient relationship. Before considering that relationship in the setting of psychiatry, we will examine several topics that relate to the problem for physicians in general.

## The Polarity of Patient and Client

PROFESSIONS AND PROFESSIONALS

The central point in much contemporary criticism of the the physician-patient relationship has to do with the conflict between autonomy and paternalism. We will treat this conflict more fully in the next chapter but wish to note here that it characterizes not only the relationship between physicians and patients, but also the dealings of all professionals with those who consult them.

There is no quintessential attribute that distinguishes professions from other occupations, but there are a number of features that, taken together, can be used to identify professional persons. A professional thus not only belongs to an occupation that demands specialized training and education; he is also expected to

exhibit a *service orientation*, to perceive the needs of . . . clients that are relevant to his competence and to attend to those needs by competent performance. [Further], in the use of his exceptional knowledge, the professional proceeds by his own judgement and authority; he thus enjoys *autonomy* restrained by responsibility.[2]

When the professional perceives certain needs in those who consult him, he may be tempted, based on his expertise, autonomy, and sense of responsibility, to decide what is best, not only in technical matters but also in ethical ones. This temptation is characteristic of all professionals, whether physicians, lawyers, teachers, clergymen, or architects, and it arises in large part because the professional's knowledge and skill are needed by people who cannot participate in the relationship as equals. As will be seen in the next chapter, professional paternalism can be judged as good or bad. What we wish to point out here is a growing concern that professionals may use their status to determine not only what is within their special competence (e.g., which operation to perform) but also what is beyond it (e.g., what loses are worth suffering as a consequence of surgery). The professional must not only be concerned with his own autonomy but also with the autonomy of those he serves.

Though the confusion of technical and ethical expertise can occur in any professional relationship, it is most dramatically seen in the practice of medicine, where the stakes may be high and the time for action short. Of late, physicians and philosophers have been struggling to redefine the physician-patient relationship and to ground it in a code of professional ethics that reflects contemporary concerns for the autonomy of the individual. One proposed solution to the problem has been to conceptualize the physician-patient relationship as contractual in nature, and it is to that approach we now turn.

THE PHYSICIAN-PATIENT RELATIONSHIP AS CONTRACT

There are, as William May notes, several potential advantages to thinking of the physician as a contractor:

First, it represents a deliberate break with more authoritarian models (such as priest or parent) for interpreting the role. At the heart of a contract is informed consent rather than blind trust; a contractual understanding of the therapeutic relationship encourages full respect for the dignity of the patient, who has not, because of illness, forfeited his sovereignty as a human being. The notion of a contract includes an exchange of information on the basis of which an agreement is reached and a subsequent exchange of goods (money for services); it also allows for a specification of rights, duties, conditions, and qualifications limiting the agreement. The net effect is to establish some symmetry and mutuality in the relationship between the doctor and the patient.

Second, a contract provides for the legal enforcement of its terms—on both parties—and thus offers both parties some protection and recourse under the law for making the other accountable for the agreement.

Finally, a contract does not rely on the pose of philanthropy, the condescension of charity. It presupposes that people are primarily governed by self-interest. When two people enter into a contract, they do so because each sees it to his own advantage.[3]

In addition to these commercial and philosophical considerations for thinking of the physician-patient relationship in contractual terms, justification can also be given on political grounds. Thus, in his argument for a contractual model of medical care, James Giles holds that the patient

should decide the issue of value-priority in the medical context. What I have been advocating is not only an ethical affirmation of the patient's right to exercise his autonomy, but a political affirmation as well. This affirmation recognizes that, in a free and democratic society, a pluralistic outcome in deciding value-priorities is inevitable. The alternative to this pluralistic vision is one that ranks values for us. This is the basis of every authoritarian political position. In its paternalistic excesses, the medical profession is often guilty of imposing, in an authoritarian manner, its value-priorities on its patients. And this occurs not because . . . the doctor represents a malevolent force, but because he wishes to help the patient and firmly believes that he possesses the expertise necessary to accomplish this end.[4]

Thus, a contractual model for the physician-patient relationship can be seen to have several potential strengths, but note must also be taken of its weaknesses. It is, for example, completely inappropriate during emergencies, in which the patient's mental or physical state makes the time-consuming and complicated procedure of negotiating a contract impossible. Though Giles believes that a contract "need not exist as a signed document" (p. 215), it is very likely that, especially in emergencies, physicians and hospitals would insist on the legal protection offered by written agreements.

But even if ways could be found to circumvent the difficulties that specific situations pose for the contractual model, it must face more general, and in our opinion, more telling criticisms. Contracts are commercial instruments, and they conduce to a commercial mentality. This type of thinking about the physician-patient relationship holds the danger of what May calls "minimalism," which reduces everything to tit for tat. Do no more for your patients than what the contract calls for. Perform specified services for certain fees and no more. The commercial contract is a fitting instrument in the purchase of an appliance, a house, or certain services that can be specified fully in advance of delivery. . . . But it would be wrong to reduce professional obligation to the specifics of a contract alone.

Professional services in the so-called helping professions are directed to subjects whose needs are in the nature of the case rather unpredictable. The professional deals with the sickness, ills, crimes, needs, and tragedies of humankind. These needs cannot be exhaustively specified in advance for each patient or client. . . . Calls upon services may be required that exceed those anticipated in a contract or for which compensation may be available in a given case. These services moreover are more likely to be effective in achieving the desired therapeutic result if they are delivered in the context of a fiduciary relationship that the patient or client can really trust.[5]

Thinking in terms of a fiduciary relationship, which is based on trust, is quite different from thinking in terms of a contractual relationship, which is based on self-interest. Indeed, the greatest threat of the contractual model to the practice of medicine is that it encourages physicians to think even more in terms of self-interest than they already do. This danger exists not only because the legal side of contracts could turn patients into potential adversaries, but also because the commercial side of contracts could turn patients into customers. In this regard it is perhaps helpful to remind those who champion the practice of calling patients *clients* that the *Oxford English Dictionary* gives this definition of *client*: "A person who employs the services of a professional or business man in any branch of business, or for whom the latter acts in his professional capacity; a customer."

Some physicians, like all people, are motivated by greed. To them, patients are customers, and their goal is to sell as many of their services as possible. These excesses might be reduced by forcing all physicians to make contracts with their patients, but it is likely that more harm than good would result.

To have "clients" or "customers" or "consumers" for one's services may seem a harmless change of nomenclature, a semantic shuffle that leaves the essence of the physician-patient relationship unchanged. It does not. The healing relationship is based on mutual trust and responsibility, and to the extent that physicians are encouraged to mistrust their patients and to avoid their professional responsibilities, to that extent the care of patients and the practice of medicine will suffer.

Though commercialism and consumerism in themselves do not necessarily lead to mistrust and irresponsibility, they may, in a paradoxical way, foster them. What physicians and patients need is not a medical ethic that forces them apart, but one that binds them together. If such an ethic cannot be found in the model of contracts, it might be found in the model of covenants.

THE PHYSICIAN-PATIENT RELATIONSHIP AS COVENANT

May has reviewed the covenantal ethic as an alternative to the contractual approach to the physician-patient relationship (pp. 67–68). He notes that the Hippocratic Oath comprises three parts: a code of duties to patients, a covenant of obligations to teachers and colleagues, and an oath to the gods of healing. The physician's obligation to his teachers and colleagues is covenantal in nature because, like biblical covenants, it begins with a debt—not to God for deliverance, but to the physician-teachers who have given him his professional life.

The gift that establishes a covenant changes one's being. As May observed,

a contract has a limited duration in time, but a covenant imposes a change on all moments. A mechanic can act under a contract, and then, when not fixing the piston, act without regard to the contract, but a covenanted people is covenanted while eating, sleeping, working, praying, stealing, cheating, healing, or blundering. . . . When the professional is initiated, he is covenanted, and the physician is a healer when he is healing, and when he is sleeping, when he is practicing, and when he is malpracticing. A covenant changes the shape of the whole life of the covenanted. (Pp. 69–70)

The covenantal obligations of physicians to their teachers and colleagues are clear in the Hippocratic Oath and in subsequent codes such as those of the American Medical Association. In these documents, "loyalty to colleagues is a responsive act for gifts already, and to be, received" (p. 70), but duties to patients are not similarly viewed.

This difference in perspective is significant because, according to May, it accounts for many of the problems with the traditional physician-patient relationship. Physicians have

thought of the patient and public as *indebted* to the profession for its services but the profession has accepted its *duties* to the patient and public out of noble conscience rather than a reciprocal sense of indebtedness.

Put another way, the medical profession imitates God not so much because it exercises power of life and death over others, but because it does not really think itself beholden, even partially, to anyone for those duties to patients which it lays upon itself. Like God, the profession draws its life from itself alone. Its action is wholly gratuitous. (P. 71)

Though we would argue with May over whether "the medical profession" takes such an attitude, we can agree with him that individual physicians do. And even if most physicians are not so arrogant, it is true that many of us take patients for granted—not our own, particular patients, but the fact that there *are* patients and that they consult us. Though it seems banal to say so, we could not be physicians without them, and we owe them a debt every bit as strong as the one we owe our teachers.

Physicians and patients are bound together by ties of reciprocal needs and satisfactions, and by promises made and kept. May stresses the role of promises in covenants by noting the difference between "descriptive" and "performative" speech. In descriptive speech

one describes a given item within the world. (It is raining. The tumor is malignant. The crisis is past.) In performative utterances, one does not merely describe a world; in effect, one alters the world by introducing an ingredient that would not be there apart from the utterance. Promises are such performative utterances. (I, John, take Thee, Mary. We will defend your country in case of attack. I will not abandon you.) . . . The doctor . . . not only tells descriptive truths, he also makes or implies promises. (I will see you next Tuesday. Despite the fact that I cannot cure you, I will not abandon you.) In brief, the moral question for the doctor is not simply a question of telling truths, but of being true to his promises. (P. 75)

Although May focuses on the performative statements of physicians, it is implied that making and keeping promises is also expected of patients. ("I will be there on Tuesday." . . . "I will take the medicine." . . . "I will tell the truth.") The sense of fidelity engendered in both parties by the keeping of promises leads to a relationship that makes curing and caring much easier. Physician and patient are "in it" together and are prepared to do things for one another that contracts are unlikely to foster.

Contracts and covenants are models for the physician-patient relationship that have their origins outside of medicine. Though much can be learned about medical practice from the perspectives of commerce, religion, politics, sociology, and philosophy, medicine exists as an institution in its own right. And though it has been influenced by the assumptions and values of other viewpoints on the human condition, it has had its own effect on what we know about ourselves, what we think is right and wrong, and what our aspirations as human beings might be.

The physician-patient relationship is a dyad. Though many other people—family members, medical colleagues, nurses, social workers, occupational therapists, technicians, dieticians, hospital administrators, insurance company employees, and government officials—are involved in it to a greater or lesser degree, the relationship between physician and patient sooner or later comes down to a "you" and a "me." This dyadic nature is not unique among professional relationships, but it does give physicians a different viewpoint from those who study the practice of medicine as nonparticipants.

The physician and patient are bound together in a common endeavor, and the study of that bond from the perspective of medicine itself must have a place in determining what society thinks a proper relationship ought to be. In this regard it is instructive to examine the views of Edmund Pellegrino, whose proposal for an ethic of medical practice begins where physicians and patients begin—with the fact of illness.

THE PHYSICIAN-PATIENT RELATIONSHIP AND THE
HEALING OF ILLNESS

Pellegrino defines illness as a subjective state in which an individual becomes anxious about his health because he has detected a change in his mental or physical functioning.[6] Illnesses may or may not be associated with demonstrable pathology, but all of them are characterized by an altered state of existence in which the person no longer believes he is "whole":

The person who becomes a patient suffers what is nothing less than an ontological assault. In our usual state we see ourselves identified with our bodies, facing the world and acting on it in essential unity. In illness the body is interposed between us and reality—it impedes our choices and actions and is no longer fully responsive. The body stands opposite to the self. Instead of serving us, we must serve it. It intrudes on our existence rather than enhancing or enriching it. (P. 44)

In this way, illness distorts the phenomenal world. The mental and physical capacities we take for granted when healthy no longer occupy the background of our thoughts and perceptions. Instead, they become the major focus of our experienced reality: "It hurts to breathe." . . . "I feel so miserable." . . . "The voices won't stop." . . . "I think I'm going to die."

Compounding the patient's distress is the knowledge that, in most cases, he cannot make himself well; that he must place his life in the hands of others; that he must suffer until he is healed.

As a physician, Pellegrino knows that when a person becomes ill he is

in an exceptionally vulnerable state, one which severely compromises his customary human freedoms to . . . make his own decisions, to act for himself, and to accept or reject the services of others. The state of being ill is therefore a state of "wounded humanity," of a person compromised in his fundamental capacity to deal with his vulnerability. (P. 45)

Being vulnerable is not unique to illness, of course, but illness confers a vulnerability that is especially threatening. That is why

healing cannot be classified as a commodity, or as a service on a par with going to a mechanic to have one's car fixed, to a lawyer for repair of one's legal fences, or even to a teacher for repair of one's defects in knowledge. The teacher-student, lawyer-client, serviceman-customer relationships have some of the elements of the physician-patient relationship. There is in them an inequality of knowledge and skill, and one person seeks assistance from another who professes to provide it. What is different is the unique ontological assault of illness on the body-self unity, and the primacy of the freedom to deal with all other life situations which illness removed. (P. 45)

It is from this special state of illness-induced vulnerability and need that Pellegrino derives the physician's obligation to use his professional knowledge and skill in the patient's interests rather than his own. The physician's responsibility is not only to be technically competent but to recognize, protect, and foster the patient's capacity to act as a moral agent:

To assure a fully participatory moral agency, the physician must repair to the extent possible the wounded humanity and state of inequality of the sick person. He does so only in part by curing, or containing, illness or relieving pain or anxiety. These must be complemented by disclosure of the information necessary for valid choice and genuine consent and by

guarding against manipulation of choice and consent to accommodate to
the physician's personal or social philosophy of the good life. (Pp. 49–50)

This is a laudable view, but physicians will recognize that in
some circumstances the patient's capacity to act as a morally autonomous agent will remain impaired unless treatment is started
and the illness relieved. This issue is a most vexing one, and we
will turn to it again in the next chapter.

Pellegrino, like May, recognizes that patients have duties of
their own if they are to be moral agents. They should, for example,
tell the truth, educate themselves about their illnesses, and not ask
their physicians to commit fraud. Indeed, Pellegrino believes that
"even though the vulnerability imposed by illness makes the patient
more vulnerable, the tyranny of the patient is as wrong as the tyranny of the physician" (p. 53).

In Pellegrino's view, neither a contract nor a covenant is an
appropriate model for the physician-patient relationship because
neither starts with the fact of illness or with an appreciation of what
it means to be a physician. Such models are more compatible with
the early Greek notion of the physician as a craftsman, but as the
the profession of medicine has developed, the craft ethic has been
modified by other forces, including the teachings of Stoic philosophers such as Panaetius, who

held that we must be faithful to the role we have assumed in life, and
that each profession has its own specific ethics. The physician has assumed a role in life that demands compassion and humaneness. These
are the physician's professional virtues. Caring, on this view, is as much
a *raison d'etre* of medicine as curing. (P. 39)

The nature of medicine and the fact of illness make it difficult
to reformulate the physician-patient relationship solely in terms of
concepts borrowed from other endeavors. What Pellegrino proposes
instead is that it be conceptualized as a "mutually binding set of
obligations, predicated upon a special kind of human interaction
and deriving its morality from the empirical realities in the relationship" (p. 53).

It is the empirical realities of physicians and patients—their
phenomenal worlds, if you will—that form the starting point for
medical practice and the healing of illness. Though different moral
principles might be used to resolve conflicts that arise in the setting
of a physician-patient relationship, it should be acknowledged that

the relationship itself is primary and that it is characterized by principles of its own.[7]

## Thinking in Terms of Psychiatric Methodology

Of all the specialties in medicine, the primacy of the physician-patient relationship is nowhere more apparent than in psychiatry. This is due both to the nature of psychiatric practice and to the fact of psychiatric illness.

Psychiatry possesses far less in the way of technology than do other specialties, so that diagnosis and treatment depend to a very great extent on the history and examination of the patient, and on the personal attributes of the physician. This is not to say that electroencephalography or blood tests or computer-assisted tomography may not be crucial in some cases, or that electroconvulsive therapy and psychopharmacology have not revolutionized psychiatric care; it is only to say that, to a degree unparalleled in contemporary medicine, the face-to-face encounter of physician and patient over time is central to the healing act. Indeed, in psychotherapy, there is nothing else; the physician-patient relationship *as a relationship* is both the vehicle and the instrument of healing.

Much of this arises from the nature of psychiatric illness. But before we can examine that issue, we must make two preliminary points. First, it should be recalled that the term *illness* refers to the patient's subjective state, while the term *disease* is a construct used by physicians to explain illnesses. Second, Pellegrino localizes the "ontological assault" of illness in the patient's body: "The body stands opposite to the self. Instead of serving us, we must serve it."[8] While this is an appropriate way of depicting many illnesses, it will not do for most psychiatric ones. In psychiatric illness, the ontological assault is not on the body but on the *self*.

We do not mean this in a categorical sense, of course, for in certain psychiatric conditions (the somatoform, depressive, and anxiety disorders, for example), bodily complaints are prominent. We also recognize that nonpsychiatric disorders are often accompanied by a change in the patient's sense of self, especially when they affect his ability to perceive, to move, or to lead a fulfilling life.

The point we wish to emphasize is that the primary abnormality in psychiatric disorders is an alteration in the patient's thinking, mood, or behavior and that these phenomena are more closely tied to his sense of self, to his essence as a person, to his existential being than are coughs, rashes, deformities, or pains. Examples of this can be found in the symptom *depersonalization*, where the very name of the phenomenon conveys a damaged sense of self, and in those syndromes characterized by delusions and hallucinations, in which the "ontological assault" may be so complete that the patient does not even realize he is ill—that he is not "himself."

The more patients are damaged in their sense of self, the less able they are to participate in contractual or covenantal relationships. Such relationships presuppose free choice, and that is exactly what persons who are "wounded" do not possess in the usual way. Illness has made them vulnerable, and therefore they need not only respect for their moral agency but also protection and understanding. Our society recognizes these needs, as the fact of involuntary hospitalization demonstrates, but, more to the point, so do psychiatrists.

If a patient who is hallucinated and delusional attacks us, we do not have him arrested. If one who is immobilized by compulsive rituals misses an appointment, we do not blame him for failing to meet the terms of a contract. And even if someone with a simple phobia—a patient barely wounded in his sense of self—refuses, through terror, to confront a phobic situation, we do not sever our bond as if he had broken a covenant.

In all of these circumstances, our actions are based on an appreciation of the patient's phenomenal world, on the fact that he is vulnerable, and on our sense of responsibility as physicians. The patient has entrusted himself to us at a time when he is not "whole," and our response to that trust is given without judging whether he is worth the effort.

Considerations such as these usually outweigh our commercial instincts—even though we are "in business"—and our political, religious, and moral beliefs, even though they are very different from those of the patient. In the context of a physician-patient relationship, much is forgiven that would otherwise be intolerable.

The call to refer to patients as *clients* can have praise-worthy motives, but it usually arises from wishful thinking—from a sentimental and superficial understanding of psychiatric disorders, and from a desire to avoid the responsibilities of a physician to those in his care. And make no mistake about it—*care*, not merely advice—is what we provide.

Care is the cement that binds physician to patient, for *care*, according to the *Oxford English Dictionary* is "Mental suffering, sorrow, grief, trouble. . . . Charge with a view to protection, preser-vation, or guidance." The patient's sense of illness is conveyed by the first definition, the physician's response—and responsibility—by the second. Though physicians can fail in that responsibility, they can also strive to meet it. After all, the watchword of medicine is still *primum non nocere*, not *caveat emptor*.

# 7

# Autonomy
# & Paternalism

When people entrust their lives to the care of physicians, they establish a relationship that can be conceptualized in a variety of ways. In this book, for example, we have so far used the polarities of Hebraic-Hellenic and patient-client to illustrate our opinion that the physician-patient relationship must be conducted in such a way that the patient's "wounded humanity" is recognized, even as his moral worth is affirmed. Here we will examine the physician's conduct in terms of another polarity—autonomy and paternalism—that speaks directly to the wish of psychiatrists to regard their patients as subject/agents who are also object/organisms.

## Suicide

THE CASE OF VIRGINIA WOOLF

Virginia Woolf was 22 years old* when she first tried to kill herself and only 59 when she succeeded in doing so. Between these attempts there was another, when she was 33, which occurred while her husband was in consultation with one of her physicians, Sir George Savage:

I was with Savage at 6.30 when I got a telephone message . . . to say that Virginia had fallen into a deep sleep. I hurried back to Brunswick

---

* Virginia Woolf's biographers disagree about the date of her initial suicide attempt. We have followed Quentin Bell's chronology, though Leonard Woolf has stated that his wife first tried to take her life at age 13.

Square and found that Virginia was lying on her bed breathing heavily and unconscious. She had taken the veronal tablets from my box and swallowed a very large dose. I telephoned to Head [a physician] and he came, bringing a nurse. Luckily Geoffrey Keynes, Maynard's brother, now Sir Geoffrey, then a young surgeon, was staying in the house. He and I got into his car and drove off as fast as we could to his hospital to get a stomach pump. . . . We drove full speed through the traffic, Geoffrey shouting to policemen that he was a surgeon 'urgent, urgent!' and they passed us through as if we were a fire engine. I do not know what time it was when we got back to Brunswick Square, but Head, Geoffrey, and the nurse were hard at work until nearly 1 o'clock in the morning. Head returned at 9 next morning (Wednesday) and said that Virginia was practically out of danger. She did not recover consciousness until the Thursday morning.[1]

Did Head, Keynes, and the nurse act appropriately? On the face of it, the question seems absurd. "Of course they did," you may be tempted to reply. "They saved her life." Ah, but that is just the point: It was *her* life and she wished to end it. Did they interfere with her *right* to do so? By preventing her death, for whatever reason, did they violate her autonomy and liberty as a human being?

IN DEFENSE OF SUICIDE

Though the defense of suicide is thought by many physicians and philosophers to be controversial,[2] some find it remarkably uncomplicated. Joseph Fletcher, for example, concluded an essay on suicide as follows:

In classical times suicide was a tragic option, for human dignity's sake. Then for centuries it was a sin. Then it became a crime. Then a sickness. Soon it will become a choice again. Suicide is the signature of freedom.[3]

The appeal of such aphorisms can be seductive, especially when the question of whether or not someone approves of suicide is made a test of whether or not he believes in freedom. It is partly for this reason that the opinions of Thomas Szasz have found an audience, especially among those who have had no clinical experience with suicidal individuals. In the following argument, for instance, Szasz explicitly identifies the prevention of suicide with totalitarianism:

It is accepted medical and psychiatric practice to treat people for their suicidal desires against their will. And what exactly does that mean? It means something quite different from the involuntary (or nonvoluntary) treatment of a bodily illness that is often given as an analogy. For a fractured ankle can be set whether or not a patient consents to its being set. It can be done because setting a fracture is a *mechanical act on the body*. But preventing suicide—suicide being the result of human desire and action—requires a *political act on the person*. In other words, since suicide is an exercise and expression of human freedom, it can be prevented only by curtailing human freedom. That is why deprivation of liberty becomes, in institutional psychiatry, a form of treatment.

In the final analysis, the would-be suicide is like the would-be emigrant: both want to leave where they are and move on elsewhere. The suicide wants to leave life and move on to death. The emigrant wants to leave his homeland and move on to another country.

Let us take the analogy seriously; after all, it is much more faithful to the facts than is the analogy between suicide and illness. A crucial characteristic that distinguishes open from closed societies is that people are free to leave the former but not the latter. The medical profession's stance on suicide is thus like the Communists' on emigration: the doctors insist that the would-be suicide survive, just as the Russians insist that the would-be emigrant stay home.[4]

Fletcher and Szasz discuss suicide in the abstract, suicide as an emblem of freedom, suicide as primarily a matter for politics and philosophy. They make it sound so easy that some wonder whether they are not correct and that the most important thing about suicide has nothing to do with the life and death of a person, but rather with abstract concepts such as autonomy and paternalism.

## The Polarity of Autonomy and Paternalism

THE TERMS DEFINED

Issues of autonomy and paternalism can be seen in almost every type of human relationship, including those of child and parent, student and teacher, patient and physician, employee and employer, and citizen and legislator. Should children be forced to attend school if they do not wish to go? Should workers be made to contribute to a retirement plan as a condition of employment? Should motorists be required to wear seat belts? These questions are quite different, but all can be answered by reference to the polarity of autonomy and paternalism.

Both terms can be defined in a number of ways, but each has a basic meaning that makes it applicable in a wide variety of circumstances. The following definitions capture that meaning and also introduce contemporary philosophers interested in the subject. Bruce Miller holds that *autonomy* "is self-determination, that the right to autonomy is the right to make one's own choices, and that respect for autonomy is the obligation not to interfere with the choice of another and to treat another as a being capable of choosing."[5]

John Kleinig's account of *paternalism* conveys his sense that the concept is best understood as a rationale for acting in a certain way toward another person: "*X* acts paternalistically in regard to *Y* to the extent that *X*, in order to secure *Y*'s good, as an end, imposes on *Y*."[6]

Miller and Kleinig are in a philosophical tradition that has struggled with the issues of autonomy and paternalism. For many, the locus classicus of that struggle is the nineteenth-century philosopher John Stuart Mill's essay *On Liberty*, in which he set forth his views on the proper relationship of the individual and society.

## ON LIBERTY

Mill's statement of his general position demonstrates his passionate concern for the rights of the individual:

The object of this Essay is to assert one very simple principle, as entitled to govern absolutely the dealings of society with the individual in the way of compulsion and control, whether the means used be physical force in the form of legal penalties, or the moral coercion of public opinion. That principle is, that the sole end for which mankind are warranted, individually or collectively, in interfering with the liberty of action of any of their number, is self-protection. That the only purpose for which power can be rightfully exercised over any member of a civilized community, against his will, is to prevent harm to others. His own good, either physical or moral, is not a sufficient warrant. He cannot rightfully be compelled to do or forbear because it will be better for him to do so, because it will make him happier, because, in the opinions of others, to do so would be wise, or even right. . . . The only part of the conduct of any one, for which he is amenable to society, is that which concerns others. In the part which merely concerns himself, his independence is, of right, absolute. Over himself, over his own body and mind, the individual is sovereign.[7]

Mill did not intend his principle to apply to everyone, however, for he immediately disqualified two groups from its scope. The first of these exclusions seems well justified:

It is, perhaps, hardly necessary to say that this doctrine is meant to apply only to human beings in the maturity of their faculties. We are not speaking of children, or of young persons below the age which the law

may fix as that of manhood or womanhood. Those who are still in a
state to require being taken care of by others, must be protected against
their own actions as well as against external injury. (P. 197)

This exclusion is important for several reasons. First, it is clear
that Mill intended society to protect those who cannot, through exercise of "mature" judgment, protect themselves. Though he men-
tions only children and "young persons," it is not unreasonable to
assume that Mill would include in this group the demented and the
severely mentally subnormal, despite the fact that they had at-
tained their legal majority.

Next, it should be noted that those in need of care may legitimately be protected against their own acts as well as against external dangers. Mill does not specify what such acts might be, but
suicide could be numbered among them without doing violence to
his concept.

Finally, the age at which children and young persons are assumed to be capable of mature judgment is entirely arbitrary, since
it is determined by the law. Society has changed its mind about
what that age should be and has also sometimes decided that different ages are approriate for "manhood or womanhood."

The second group that Mill immediately excluded from his doctrine makes it even more evident that the age of an individual is
not the only factor to be weighed when deciding whether or not that
person possesses mature faculties:

For the same reason, we may leave out of consideration those backward
states of society in which the race itself may be considered as in its non-
age. The early difficulties in the way of spontaneous progress are so
great, that there is seldom any choice of means for overcoming them;
and a ruler full of the spirit of improvement is warranted in the use of
any expedients that will attain an end, perhaps otherwise unattainable.
Despotism is a legitimate mode of government in dealing with barbari-
ans, provided the end be their improvement, and the means justified by
actually effecting that end. Liberty, as a principle, has no application to
any state of things anterior to the time when mankind have become capable of being improved by free and equal discussion. (Pp. 197–98)

There are many things that could be said about this passage,
but the point we wish to emphasize here is that even adults may
have certain decisions made for them if they are unable to participate in "free and equal discussion," provided the intervention can
be defended as beneficial in the long run.

Later in *On Liberty*, Mill noted a third exception to his principle that the individual is sovereign over his own body and mind, an exception that bears more directly on the issue of suicide:

In this and most other civilized countries . . . an engagement by which a person should sell himself, or allow himself to be sold, as a slave, would be null and void; neither enforced by law nor by opinion. The ground for thus limiting his power of voluntarily disposing of his own lot in life, is apparent, and is very clearly seen in this extreme case. The reason for not interfering, unless for the sake of others, with a person's voluntary acts, is consideration for his liberty. His voluntary choice is evidence that what he so chooses is desirable, or at the least endurable, to him, and his good is on the whole best provided for by allowing him to take his own means of pursuing it. But by selling himself for a slave, he abdicates his liberty; he forgoes any future use of it, beyond that single act. (P. 304)

The application of Mill's doctrine is further complicated by his acknowledgment that people are bound to one another in a variety of ways—that few important acts are "self-regarding" in the sense that they are of concern only to the actor:

No person is an entirely isolated being; it is impossible for a person to do anything seriously or permanently hurtful to himself, without mischief reaching at least to his near connections, and often far beyond them. . . . When, by conduct of this sort, a person is led to violate a distinct and assignable obligation to any other person or persons, the case is taken out of the self-regarding class. . . . Whenever, in short, there is a definite damage, or a definite risk of damage, either to an individual or to the public, the case is taken out of the province of liberty, and placed in that of morality or law. (Pp. 277–79)

Mill's acknowledgment of the responsibilities we bear one another has clear implications for the issue of suicide. A further example of this concern for the interrelatedness of people and its modifying effect on the doctrine of non-interference is seen in the following passage, which has special relevance for the physician's role in suicide prevention:

There are also many positive acts for the benefit of others, which [an individual] may rightfully be compelled to perform; such as, to give evidence in a court of justice; to bear his fair share in the common defence . . . and to perform certain acts of individual beneficence, such as saving a fellow creature's life, or interposing to protect the defenceless against ill-usage, things which whenever it is obviously a man's duty to do, he may rightfully be made responsible to society for not doing. A person may cause evil to others not only by his actions but by his inaction, and in either case he is justly accountable to them for the injury. (Pp. 198–99)

These exceptions and qualifications to Mill's principle demonstrate that he believed well-meaning interventions could be warranted in certain circumstances. Though *On Liberty* is often cited in defense of autonomy, it is clear that the essay can also be adduced in support of paternalism.

The tension between autonomy and paternalism found in works of political philosophy such as *On Liberty* is also seen in the writings of physicians and philosophers interested in medical ethics and the physician-patient relationship. In the following section we will review some aspects of the conflict between autonomy and paternalism that relate to the practice of medicine in general.

### Autonomy, Paternalism, and the Practice of Medicine

In one of the first papers in the medical literature to address the issue of autonomy and paternalism specifically, Thomas Szasz and Marc Hollender propose three models of the physician-patient relationship: activity-passivity; guidance-cooperation; and mutual participation.[8] Each model is considered appropriate in particular clinical situations, and each is seen as the expression of a more basic type of human relationship.

Patients in shock or coma, for example, are unable to contribute to their own care, so that, for them, the activity-passivity model is thought most suitable. In this type of relationship, according to Szasz and Hollender, there is a similarity "between the patient and a helpless infant, on the one hand, and between the physician and a parent, on the other" (p. 586).

For patients who are acutely ill, but conscious and able to participate in their own treatment, the guidance-cooperation model is fitting. The physician is again likened by Szasz and Hollender to a parent because of his knowledge and power, while the patient is seen as an adolescent child, who, though possessing power of his own, is expected "neither to question nor to argue or disagree with the orders he receives" (p. 587).

Their final model of the physician-patient relationship, mutual participation, is exemplified by chronic conditions in which the physician's major responsibility is to help the patient to help himself. Here, the participants are seen as interdependent adults of approximately equal power.

Szasz and Hollender note that, over time, a particular physician-patient relationship may be characterized by all three models, as the clinical situation moves from diabetic coma to mild diabetic ketoacidosis to well-controlled diabetes, for example, and that problems can arise if the physician-parent does not realize the emerging needs of the patient-child for a greater sense of equality.

As they seek to identify good medical practice from the viewpoint of human relationships, Szasz and Hollender propose a source of trouble that may often be overlooked: a mismatch in the expectations physicians and patients can have of one another over issues of autonomy and paternalism. This focus could explain their discussion of relationships primarily in terms of power rather than trust, affection, sharing, or other themes that characterize human interactions, including those between physicians and patients. But it also may be, as they ask what constitutes "good medicine," that Szasz and Hollender touch on an issue that has grown increasingly important in the last several decades: Who decides what is best?

Who decides what is best has, in some instances, become a question of power, at least as power is reflected in the judgments of courts, the decisions of review boards, and the actions of legislators. Should large amounts of public monies be spent to help a small number of patients with a rare disease? How is it decided who receives treatment when facilities are limited? Should patients be allowed to die? Should they be helped to die? Vexing questions like these lead not only to a consideration of what constitutes "good medicine" but also to an examination of the purpose of medicine in the contemporary world.

THE PURPOSE OF MEDICINE

In the view of Eric Cassell, the basic goal of medicine should be to preserve the patient's autonomy in deciding what is best.[9] Before examining his argument, however, we must return for a moment to the concept of autonomy itself. Philosophers interested in the polarity of autonomy and paternalism[10] have agreed that acts cannot be considered truly autonomous unless they are "authentic." Someone acts authentically when he acts "himself"—when his conduct reflects his characteristic attitudes, beliefs, intentions, and values.

Cassell accepts this point and, following Gerald Dworkin, also argues that the concept of autonomy requires "independence" of action. Independence, for Cassell, is freedom of choice, which, to be meaningful, must be based on knowledge of the area in which the choice is to be made, on the ability to think clearly, and on the capacity to act effectively.

In Cassell's opinion, it is the illness, not the physician, that deprives the patient of his authenticity and independence and thus robs him of his autonomy:

Am I my authentic self when I am foul-smelling from vomitus or feces, lying in the mess of my illness? . . . Is that my authentic father lying there, hooked up to tubes and wires, weak and powerless? It is clear that illness can impair authenticity.

But if illness has an effect on authenticity, what does it do to independence? If freedom of choice requires knowledge, then the sick do not have the same freedom of choice as the well. Knowledge, for the sick person, is incomplete and (for the very sick) never can be complete even if the patient is a physician. . . .

Not only is knowledge lacking for the sick person but reason is also impaired. In the simplest terms, it is difficult to be clear headed in pain or suffering. . . . The final element necessary for meaningful free choice is the ability to act. Illness so obviously interferes with the ability to act as to require almost no comment.[11]

Here Cassell, like Pellegrino, appreciates that illness is an "ontological assault" on the patient, that it severely distorts his phenomenal world, and that it alters his relationships with others:

It is reasonable to conclude that illness interferes with autonomy to a degree dependent on the nature and severity of the illness, the person involved, and the setting. The sick person is deprived of wholeness by the loss of complete independence and by the loss of complete authenticity. What helps restore wholeness? It should first be pointed out that autonomy is a relational term. Autonomy is exercised in relation to others; it is encouraged or defeated by the action of others as well as by the actor. For this reason wholeness can be restored to the sick (in terms of autonomy) in part by family and friends. However, there are limits to the capacity of family or friends in returning autonomy to the sick . . . [for] they, like he, cannot act against the most important thief of autonomy, the illness.

There is one relationship from which wholeness can be returned to the patient and that is the relationship with the doctor. The doctor-patient relationship can be the source from which both authenticity and independence can be returned to the patient. The degree of restoration will depend on both patient and doctor and is subject to the limits imposed by the disease. *I am also well aware that by his actions or lack of them, the physician can further destroy rather than repair the patient's au-*

*tonomy. But here I am not speaking of what harm can be done but what
good can be done.* (Pp. 41–42)

If the physician is the only one who can restore the patient's
autonomy in certain circumstances, there is a place for paternalism
in the practice of "good medicine." And though physicians must acknowledge that they sometimes deprive patients of autonomy
through an unreflective use of power (a point Szasz and Hollender
wish to make), it is also true that failure to accept responsibility
for relieving the patient's "wounded humanity" can perpetuate his
illness and thus his dependent state. Indeed, Mark Komrad proposes
that a reciprocal interaction between autonomy and paternalism is
the only defensible basis for the physician-patient relationship.[12]

Komrad argues that illness and the sick role that accompanies
it represent a state of diminished autonomy. Medical paternalism
should be understood as a response to that state rather than as a
negation of the patient's rights:

When seen in this way—as a special kind of diminished autonomy—the
sick role naturally invites the physician to behave paternally [i.e., at the
patient's request] if not frankly paternalistically, to fill the void left as
autonomy diminishes. Incidentally, one would not want the physician to
behave in any other way since paternalism is the only type of response
that properly puts the patient's good above all other considerations. According to this view, some paternalism is not only justified but is required in all therapeutic relationships due to the nature of illness and
the sick role. Paternalism is not always incompatible with the principle
of autonomy and, in fact, paternalism may be instituted to preserve autonomy (as in Mill's slavery example) to restore it (as in the doctor-patient relationship), or to establish it (as in paternalism towards children). The restitution of diminished autonomy is the only rationalisation
of medical paternalism that does not profane autonomy. The admonition
that a physician should "respect the patient's autonomy" does not explicitly acknowledge that a patient presents in a condition of incomplete autonomy. Rather, one might more appropriately ask instead that the doctor respect the patient's *potential for autonomy*. The maximisation of
autonomy within the bounds of the patient's potential seems to me a legitimate goal of the therapeutic encounter. (Pp. 41–42)

It is important to note that, in all of the arguments for limited
paternalism in medical practice we have reviewed, the patient's experience of illness, with all its pain, anxiety, helplessness, impa-
tience, and bewilderment, is clearly appreciated. We emphasize this
point because, in some discussions of the polarity of autonomy and

paternalism, it may seem that "rights" and "power" are the only things involved. As Cassell put it:

When philosophers and lawyers (and many others) talk about rights they often speak as though the body does not exist. When they discuss the rights of patients they act as if a sick person is simply a well person with an illness appended. Like putting on a knapsack, the illness is added but nothing else changes. That is simply a wrong view of the sick.[13]

Such insensitivity to suffering may occur through lack of clinical experience or because a political/economic perspective on the practice of medicine does not discern patients and physicians except as metaphors for something else. If this can happen with illnesses primarily involving "the body" and that are manifest by signs as obvious as cough, deformity, and wasting, imagine how much more difficult it may be for philosophers and lawyers (and many physicians) to appreciate "the fact of illness" when the patient's body seems whole—when his illness is manifest primarily in his thoughts, moods, and behaviors. The problem here is not that rights are discussed as if "the mind" did not exist, but rather as if mental life could never be abnormal, as if all thoughts were "authentic," all moods were "understandable," and all acts not coerced by others were "independent." These issues are nowhere more apparent in the practice of medicine than in the matter of suicide.

## Thinking in Terms of Psychiatric Methodology

THE PHENOMENON OF SUICIDE

Some who hold that physicians should not intervene in suicide reason in terms of the following syllogism: Physicians treat diseases; suicide is not a disease; therefore, physicians who prevent suicide are not acting as physicians when they do so—since there is nothing to "treat"—but as ordinary citizens, who can legitimately be held responsible for assaulting the person they are trying to "help." Though we would dispute the major premise (because physicians have always treated *illnesses*, even when no bodily pathology has been, or could be, demonstrated), we are in complete agreement with the minor premise: suicide is not a disease. We do not, however, take the truth of this statement as an argument that physicians have no role in suicide prevention; rather, we take it as evidence that the nature of suicide has not been understood.

Suicide is not a disease or an illness but a behavior, an activity designated by its consequences. To make this point, we will first illustrate the concept of behaviors with an activity that is much less controversial than suicide, eating:

Human beings employ many coordinations of hand, eye, and mouth, but we recognize and distinguish among them the behavior of eating, in which the activity leads to the consequence of food consumption. Eating is a clear and specific behavior, even though its particular appearance on any occasion may vary depending on the state of the organism, the availability of nutrients, personal attitudes toward food, and social custom. Yet even though the behavior can be performed under differing circumstances and can be disturbed in certain ways (for example, overeating, undereating, pica), it is clear that we are always considering manifestations of the same phenomenon—the behavior of eating—and that an understanding of the behavior, whether normal or abnormal, must consider issues ranging from the biological to the cultural.[14]

In the same way, human beings have many activities involving pills, guns, knives, ropes, and automobiles, but we can distinguish among them the behavior of suicide, in which the intended consequence is the death of the actor. We are not speaking here of self-injury for other purposes, which can include the ritual skin incisions of a culturally sanctioned ceremony, the attention-seeking minor overdose of an impulsive and self-dramatizing person, and the carefully planned symbolic self-mutilation of someone responding to the commands of hallucinated voices. In none of these behaviors is death the goal, though it may occur through ignorance or mischance. What we will discuss is suicide—that self-injury whose aim is death—because it brings into sharp focus the polarity of autonomy and paternalism in the practice of medicine and psychiatry.

To identify suicide as a behavior is also to acknowledge that, like other behaviors, it can be associated with a variety of phenomena. One may engage in the behavior of eating, for example, because one is hungry, or bored, or waiting for a friend in the cafeteria; or because one writes a column on restaurants and has a deadline to meet; or because one has a delusional belief that particular foods must be consumed at a certain time, lest the world be destroyed. All of these are possible reasons for the behavior of eating, but they are not equally common ones. To learn about eating in its most frequent form, one would study the relationship of that behavior to the phenomenon of hunger.

So, too, with the behavior of suicide. One may attempt to kill oneself because one is delusionally hopeless in the setting of a depressive disorder; or because one is a soldier about to be captured by a cruel enemy; or because one has a painful terminal illness; or because one wishes to make a dramatic political statement; or because one is prohibited from marrying one's beloved. All of these are possible reasons for suicide, and to read many of the philosophical, literary, and political writings on the subject, one could think they were equally frequent. If such writings deal with the epidemiology of suicide at all, it is only in terms of opinions or guesses and almost never in terms of data, perhaps because data are considered irrelevant when a meaningful idea is being defended. For physicians, it is usually foolish to base one's practice on rare cases or, even worse, on hypothetical ones. Before one can speak with confidence about suicide, one should know not only what kind of phenomenon it is but also what kind of phenomena it is most often associated with.

SUICIDE: SOME FACTS

In order to provide information about suicide that is useful to physicians faced with the decision of whether or not they should intervene to prevent it, studies must examine the characteristics of individuals who are representative of the behavior. Though the dishonored samurai warrior who commits *seppuku* and the patient with terminal amyotrophic lateral sclerosis who unplugs his respirator both teach us something about suicide, they may not be the best examples on which to base our decisions about the behavior. Physicians must know the circumstances in which the majority of suicides occur, since, if illness is involved, physicians may be called upon to act.

The two studies we will mention in this section describe representative samples of suicidal individuals. They deal with people who had actually killed themselves, rather than those who had attempted to do so but survived or those who had injured themselves for other purposes. Such research is retrospective in nature but has the advantage of examining the characteristics of people in whom the motivation to die was likely to have been strong.

Both studies set out to discover what proportion of suicidal individuals had suffered from mental disorders before their deaths. The investigators were explicitly concerned with methodological issues such as the quality and quantity of information available to them, the reliability and validity of their diagnoses, and the relationship of their findings to the work of other researchers. Though the two studies were carried out in countries with different procedures for establishing death by suicide, and though the two groups of investigators had been trained in different traditions of psychiatric diagnosis, their findings were quite similar.

Thus, in a study of 100 English suicides by Brian Barraclough and his colleagues,[15] 93 percent were identified as having been mentally ill before their deaths. The most frequent diagnosis, made in 70 percent of cases, was depressive disorder. This diagnosis did not rest on the fact of suicide itself but on the recognition of a pattern of signs and symptoms that was similar to (if more severe than) that found in an unselected sample of depressed patients from the same community.

The next most common diagnosis made by Barraclough et al. was alcoholism, which was identified in 15 percent of cases. The alcohol abuse by this group of suicides tended to be chronic and severe, with nearly all of them having experienced convulsions, delirium tremens, or permanent memory loss. In addition, many depressive symptoms were recorded, so that over half of the group was given a diagnosis of depression in addition to that of alcoholism.

Eight of the 15 remaining suicides were felt to have had a variety of psychiatric conditions, and in seven cases a diagnosis of mental illness was not made. In this last group, however, the investigators were often uncertain as to whether or not a diagnosis was warranted because, as the case histories summarized in the paper indicate, a depressive disorder was possible or likely in several instances.

In the second study we wish to review, Eli Robins reported on 134 unselected suicides in the city of St. Louis and St. Louis County.[16] The diagnostic criteria employed are given in detail, as are summaries for each of the 134 cases. Ninety-four percent of the suicides studied were diagnosed as having had a psychiatric disorder before their deaths, while 4 percent had suffered with terminal medical illnesses, and 2 percent had apparently been well.

Like Barraclough et al., Robins found that depression and alcoholism accounted for most of the psychiatric diagnoses made. Thus, in cases where a diagnosis could be given with confidence, 47 percent of suicides were believed to have been depressed and 25 percent to have been alcoholics. Fifteen percent of the 134 cases were felt to have had some type of psychiatric disorder, though the information available was insufficient to permit specific diagnoses to be made. If it is assumed that the proportion of depressed and alcoholic individuals was the same in this ill-but-undiagnosed group as it was among other cases, the two conditions would account for 82 percent of the total diagnoses made, as compared with the 85 percent rate found by Barraclough et al.

It is to be noted that, even though depression and alcoholism can be recognized in the great majority of individuals who commit suicide, most people with these illnesses never take their lives. Other factors, such as male sex, increasing age, and social isolation have repeatedly been shown (as they were by Robins and by Barraclough et al.) to increase the risk for suicide, though presumably they exert their effects on individuals who are already more vulnerable to that behavior because of affective disorder, alcohol abuse, and other psychiatric illnesses.

That a variety of factors has been found to influence the decision to commit suicide is not surprising; indeed, it is expected. Suicide is a behavior, and as such, its occurrence and its expression are shaped by phenomena ranging from the biological to the cultural. What is important to acknowledge in a discussion of autonomy and paternalism, however, is that all of these phenomena should not be given equal weight in the equation of death. As Barraclough and his colleagues observed: "Mental illness is an essential component of suicide; our findings . . . suggest that in Western society suicide in the healthy person is a rare event."[17]

SUICIDE AND AUTONOMY

If the behavior of suicide is almost always associated with psychiatric illness, it is likely that the decision to take one's life is neither authentic nor independent and therefore hardly autonomous. Authenticity and independence require that the phenomenal world be intact, and in depressive disorders, alcoholism, and the other psychiatric conditions associated with suicide, the phenomenal world is severely distorted. We do not mean here that autonomous decisions can *never* be made in the setting of *any* illness, but only that the more an illness disturbs the phenomenal world, the less likely the patient is to act authentically and independently.

Independence, according to Cassell,[18] rests in part on clear thinking. To the extent that alcoholics, for example, are unable to think clearly because of intoxication, hallucinosis, delirium tremens, Korsakoff's syndrome, or dementia, to that extent they are unable to act independently.

Authenticity, or acting oneself, can also be diminished by the psychiatric disorders that predispose to suicide. If, as in many depressive illnesses, the phenomenal world is altered by delusions, the actions based on those false beliefs will be inauthentic. Inauthenticity can be recognized not only in behavior (such as suicide) that is completely alien to the individual but also (and more commonly) in delusional distortions of familiar characteristics. An example of this latter type of inauthenticity is found in Leonard Woolf's description of his wife's attitude to eating and how it was affected by her manic-depressive illness:

In the first weeks at Dalingridge the most difficult and distressing problem was to get Virginia to eat. If left to herself, she would have eaten nothing at all and would have gradually starved to death. Here again her psychology and behaviour were only a violent exaggeration of what they were when she was well and sane. When she was well, she was essentially a happy and gay person; she enjoyed the ordinary things of everyday life, and among them food and drink. Yet there was always something strange, something slightly irrational in her attitude towards food. It was extraordinarily difficult ever to get her to eat enough to keep her strong and well. Superficially I suppose it might have been said that she had a (quite unnecessary) fear of becoming fat; but there was something deeper than that, at the back of her mind or in the pit of her stomach a taboo against eating. Pervading her insanity generally there was always a sense of some guilt, the origin and exact nature of which I could never discover; but it was attached in some peculiar way particularly to food and eating. In the early acute, suicidal stage of the depression, she would sit for hours overwhelmed with hopeless melancholia, silent, making no response to anything said to her. When the time for a meal came, she would pay no attention whatsoever to the plate of food put before her and, if the nurses tried to get her to eat something, she became enraged. I could usually induce her to eat a certain amount, but it was a terrible process. . . .

This excruciating business of food, among other things, taught me a lesson about insanity which I found it very difficult to learn—it is useless to argue with an insane person. . . . In ordinary life, as her writings, and particularly her essays, show, Virginia had an extraordinarily clear and logical mind. . . . There were moments or periods during her illness, particularly in the second excited stage, when she was what could be called "raving mad" and her thoughts and speech became completely unco-ordinated, and she had no contact with reality. Except for these periods, she remained all through her illness, even when most insane, terribly sane in three-quarters of her mind. The point is that her insanity was in her premises, in her beliefs. She believed, for instance, that she was not ill, that her symptoms were due to her own "faults". . . that the doctors and nurses were in conspiracy against her. These beliefs were insane because they were in fact contradicted by reality. But given these beliefs as premises for conclusions and actions, all Virginia's actions and conclusions were logical and rational; and her power of arguing conclusively from false premises was terrific. It was therefore useless to attempt to argue with her . . . about what you wanted her to do, e.g. eat her breakfast, because if her premises were true, she could prove and did prove conclusively to you that she ought not to eat her breakfast.[19]

But in the case of Virginia Woolf, there is an even more dramatic illustration of the inauthenticity brought about by her illness: between her first and second suicide attempts, there was an interval of 11 years; and between her second and third attempts, an interval of 26 years. The authentic Virginia Woolf did not want to die.

THE PHYSICIAN'S RESPONSIBILITY

If the effect of illness is to rob people of autonomy and the function of medicine is to preserve or restore that autonomy, then the responsibility of physicians to suicidal patients is clear. If it is incompatible with the principle of liberty that one should be permitted to sell himself into slavery, then it is incompatible with the principle of autonomy that one should be permitted to take his life. Whether the issue is liberty or autonomy, he who deprives himself of it "forgoes any future use of it, beyond that single act."

Though discussions of autonomy and paternalism may be pursued in the abstract and at leisure, the practice of medicine requires decisions by real people in real time. Some principle, some rule of thumb, should inform these decisions, and the one we propose is the following: Treat every suicide attempt as the inauthentic action of an individual who has been deprived of his autonomy by illness.

This principle has several advantages. First, it is likely to be correct, since the overwhelming majority of people who kill themselves are ill. If the illness can be reversed, autonomy can be restored. Next, it obviates the need to distinguish in emergencies between acts whose goal is self-dramatization and acts whose goal is self-destruction. In both instances the amount of damage produced may be small, but in the case of the truly suicidal individual, little harm may be done only because he has miscalculated or is making a "trial run." Finally, the principle recognizes that people exist in a web of relationships, that suicide is never entirely "self-regarding," and that the physician's obligation is to remember others, even if the patient cannot.

Our principle is not meant to govern the physician's conduct in all conceivable situations; it is intended as a rule of thumb, not an edict. In certain circumstances, to insist on life at any cost may be as lacking in compassion as to insist on death at any time. But these situations are likely to be rare, and decisions regarding them should be reached only after much reflection and consultation.

There are also undoubtedly circumstances in which the principle would be mistakenly applied, thereby depriving someone of his autonomy or liberty without adequate justification. Fortunately, there are ways to reverse such decisions, though the same cannot usually be said of death.

A QUESTION OF PERSPECTIVES

The perspective of psychiatry on suicide is quite different from that of philosophy or the law. Though such disciplines share with medicine a vital interest in the polarity of autonomy and paternalism as it relates to issues of life and death, their viewpoints are not clinical ones, and their practitioners are without responsibility, save that owed by one human being to another.

We do not mean here that only psychiatrists are qualified to speak on suicide, or that the practice of medicine should not be judged except by its own standards. Decisions about life and death are properly the concern of all institutions whose task it is to clarify moral issues. What we do insist upon, however, is that psychiatry provides information about suicide that is unavailable from other sources and that such information is essential to an understanding of the phenomenon.

From the viewpoint of the clinic, suicide is not only a behavior with a certain epidemiology; it is also an act filled with meaning. Suicidal individuals can be counted, but they are more than statistics. To the suicide, and to those who know and care for him, the meanings of his death are almost never experienced in terms of autonomy and paternalism but rather in painful emotions such as despair, anger, and bewilderment. The meaning of suicide may, of course, be taken as "the signature of freedom," but only through a kind of moral inversion in which abstract ideas become more important than individual suffering.

Once it is granted that psychiatrists and other physicians have a legitimate role in understanding suicidal behavior, there are still problems caused by differences in perspective. If, for example, suicide is considered only in terms of the life-story method, it will always be regarded as the meaningful choice of a troubled self. From this perspective, psychotherapy will be deemed the only appropriate treatment, and, should it fail, the poor outcome will be attributed to the patient's resistance or to the therapist's lack of skill. If, however, suicide is thought of only as the manifestation of conditions, like manic-depressive disorder, best explained from the perspective of the disease concept, medications and electroconvulsive therapy will be prescribed, and, should they fail, the poor outcome will be attributed to inadequate drug levels or to the refractoriness of the disorder.

The problem here is not that one perspective is inherently right and the other wrong, but that each has been used as if it were the only construct necessary for an understanding of suicide. Once suicide is seen as a behavior, the antagonism between defenders of life stories and diseases, minds and brains, agents and organisms, is resolved, for all of these concepts are necessary to understand the phenomenon. And since the most appropriate treatment of suicidal behavior depends on what it is associated with, the choice of psychotherapy and/or pharmacotherapy becomes a matter for differential diagnosis rather than for dogma.

THE CASE OF VIRGINIA WOOLF

Though the story of Virginia Woolf's life is an extraordinary one, the story of her death is all too common. She suffered from manic-depressive disorder, a condition that shaped her development as a person and as a writer, affected her closest relationships, and eventually claimed her life.

As her husband noted, for many years her family, friends, and physicians cared for and protected her through bouts of illness they did not understand and could not interrupt:

I do not know what the present state of knowledge with regard to nervous and mental diseases is in the year 1963; in 1913 it was desperately meagre. . . . Over the years I consulted five neurologists or mental specialists, all at the head of their profession. . . . They were all men of the highest principle and good will; they were all (or had been) brilliant doctors; I have no doubt that they knew as much about the human mind and its illnesses as any of their contemporaries. It may sound arrogant on my part when I say that it seemed to me that what they knew amounted to practically nothing. They had not the slightest idea of the nature or the cause of Virginia's mental state, which resulted in her suddenly or gradually losing touch with the real world, so that she lived in a world of delusions and became a danger to herself and other people. Not knowing how or why this had happened to her, naturally they had no real or scientific knowledge of how to cure her. All they could say was that she was suffering from neurasthenia and that, if she could be induced or compelled to rest and eat and if she could be prevented from committing suicide, she would recover. (Pp. 159–60)

Because she was "induced," "compelled," and "prevented"—because others intervened in a paternalistic way—Virginia Woolf always did recover, with her autonomy restored, until the final illness.

As for the state of knowledge with regard to manic-depressive disorder in 1986, our ability to diagnose and treat it is much improved, though an explanation of its etiology is still lacking. The physicians who attended Virginia Woolf may have misidentified her condition, but they knew that suicide was a risk and that recovery was the rule. Virginia Woolf always did recover and, in the intervals, became her authentic self. If she had been saved after her last suicide attempt, at age 59, she might well have come to write what she did after her first, at age 22:

Oh my Violet, if there were a God I should bless him for having delivered me safe and sound from the miseries of the last six months! You cant think what an exquisite joy every minute of my life is to me now, and my only prayer is that I may live to be 70.[20]

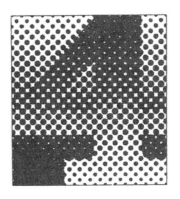

# *Conclusion*

# 8

# The Ambiguity
# of Psychiatry:
# A Methodological
# Resolution

Psychiatry can be ambiguous because, as Jaspers observed, human nature is ambiguous:

> The human being is not merely a kind of animal nor is he any kind of purely spiritual creature of which we have no knowledge and which earlier times conceived to be angelic. Man is rather something *unique*; he partakes in the series of *living things* and in the series of *angel*, belonging to both and differing from both.[1]

The ambiguity of human nature is seen by physicians only in psychiatry's domain—the phemonenal world—for it is only there that the animal and spiritual aspects of the human self are both evident. Indeed, the phenomenal world is the locus of *all* human distress, whether caused by disease of the body or anguish of the soul, whether by disorder of the brain or disturbance of the mind, for it is only in the phenomenal world that illness is experienced and expressed, only there that it is communicated and comprehended.

Since the self can neither be constructed from the animal brain up nor derived from the spiritual mind down, it is pointless trying to turn psychiatry either into one of the physical sciences or one of the humanities. Though both explanation and understanding are necessary in psychiatry, neither is sufficient for a discipline that must deal in a practical way with the ambiguity of human nature and human illness.

George Engel has also struggled with this problem, and has turned to general systems theory as an integrating concept.[2] The "biopsychosocial model" he proposed has reminded psychiatrists of the need for considering multiple levels of information as they make clinical and theoretical formulations.

We agree that information must be derived from many different levels for the best practice of psychiatry, but more than information is required. The biopsychosocial approach does not synthesize information into a coherent formulation; it does not generate a sequence of reasoning whose boundaries or directions are clear. Engel's model lists the ingredients but does not provide the recipe.

In *The Perspectives of Psychiatry*,[3] we tried to demonstrate the value of thinking about disorders in terms of four distinct constructs: diseases, dimensions of human variation, behaviors, and the life stories of selves choosing to live one way rather than another. Each of these perspectives illuminates aspects of the phenomenal world, but none can see it all. To assert dogmatically that any single viewpoint defines the field of psychiatry (rather than the fields of neuroscience, behaviorism, or psychoanalysis, for example) is to miss both the essence and the ambiguity of the self.

Yet a call for multiple perspectives in psychiatry should not be interpreted as a call for unreflective eclecticism, a kind of methodological porridge in which all ideas are considered equivalent. Eclecticism of that sort tends to misunderstand and to underestimate the conceptual impediments to a unification of thought in psychiatry and seems callow in its happy suggestion that we need only judge ideas from their practical results and accept "whatever works." Such eclecticism ignores the fact that the perspectives of psychiatry are rule governed, that behind each, whether we know it or not, is a structure that generates a particular set of observations, interpretations, and expectations.

Psychiatrists must decide how to elucidate a disorder such as schizophrenia, for example. It may seem to the eclectic that a decision of this type is simply a matter of choosing from among equivalent opinions, that it is a question of personal preference, of what "you feel most comfortable with." In fact, psychiatric choices are derived from radically different conceptual perspectives—diseases, dimensions, behaviors, and life stories—each of which has its own set of expectations and rules of procedure. These rules and expectations have an insistent power as they direct our inquiry in one direction rather than another, an insistence that produces ignorance—if not rejection—of alternative perspectives with different rules and expectations.

The monopolistic tendency of each perspective rests on the persuasive promise of any unity of vision. The psychoanalytic psychiatrist sees that the life-story perspective is a powerful one and that its ability to account for distress will increase as basic human motivations and conflicts are better discerned. The neuropsychiatrist, on the other hand, sees that the concept of brain pathology is in its explanatory infancy and that advances in neuroscience will place more and more psychiatric conditions within the perspective of disease. It is not just what they can do that differentiates these perspectives, it is what axioms they assume, what rules they follow, and what promises they make.

These generative features will always exist within each perspective, and no amount of well-intentioned ignoring of them can gloss over their implications. It is thus more than a question of taste whether we think about schizophrenia as a clinical syndrome whose pathophysiology and etiology will be revealed through the application of the disease concept; as an extreme deviation along a dimension of psychological development that ranges from normal through neurotic and "borderline" to psychotic; as a set of maladaptive behaviors, a cluster of bad habits that must be unlearned; or as an "alternative life style," the understandable response of a sensitive person to an "insane" family or culture.

Each of these proposals makes different assumptions about the phenomenal world and its disorders, and each has different consequences for psychiatric practice and research. To hold that it makes no difference which of them we use is to adopt "the comfortable posture of those who wish to offend no one, even at the risk of satisfying no one."[4] Indeed, the result of ignoring the fundamental differences between perspectives is not to diminish sectarianism but, in the end, to encourage it.

We can accept neither a bellicose denominationalism nor an unreflective eclecticism. The former brings confidence at the price of blindness; the latter, breadth at the cost of naïveté. What will give us both sureness and scope in the face of psychiatry's inherent ambiguity is an approach that acknowledges the several perspectives in the field and yet maintains a critical stance toward each of them, an approach that encourages questions like, "What is there about schizophrenia that leads us to think that the construct of diseases is more likely to be helpful in revealing the disorder's cause than are the constructs of dimensions, behaviors, and life stories?" and "What harmful consequences could arise if the disease construct

were misapplied; if it were thought just as appropriate for demoralization as it seems to be for schizophrenia?" Such a stance encourages debate but acknowledges that standards exist whereby debate can be ended—standards that are not derived from sectarian
allegiance or naïve relativism, but from an appreciation that all
claims suppose a method and that all methods limit our vision in
particular ways. Psychiatry's ambiguity and multiple perspectives
demand that we be broad-minded and tough-minded, but above all
they demand that we be clearheaded.

# Notes

Chapter 1. Psychiatry's Domain

1. Paul R. McHugh and Phillip R. Slavney, *The Perspectives of Psychiatry* (Baltimore: Johns Hopkins University Press, 1983).
2. Wolfgang Köhler, *Gestalt Psychology* (New York: Horace Liveright, 1929), pp. 3–4.
3. Michael Alan Schwartz and Osborne Wiggins, "Science, Humanism, and the Nature of Medical Practice: A Phenomenological View," *Perspectives in Biology and Medicine* 28 (1985): 331–61.

Chapter 2. Mind & Brain

1. Colin Murray Parkes, *Bereavement: Studies of Grief in Adult Life* (New York: International Universities Press, 1972), p. 39.
2. John Bowlby, *Attachment and Loss*, 3 vols. (New York: Basic Books, 1969–80), 3: 94.
3. John Bowlby, "Processes of Mourning," *International Journal of Psycho-Analysis* 42 (1961): 317–40; William T. McKinney, Jr. and William E. Bunney, Jr., "Animal Model of Depression: I. Review of Evidence: Implications for Research," *Archives of General Psychiatry* 21 (1969): 240–48; and Kathlyn L. R. Rasmussen and Martin Reite, "Loss-Induced Depression in an Adult Macaque Monkey," *American Journal of Psychiatry* 139 (1982): 679–81.
4. Sigmund Freud, "Mourning and Melancholia," in *The Standard Edition of the Complete Psychological Works of Sigmund Freud*, trans. and ed. James Strachey, 24 vols. (London: Hogarth Press and the Institute of Psycho-Analysis, 1953–74), 14: 243–58, and Paula J. Clayton, James A. Halikas, and William L. Maurice, "The Depression of Widowhood," *British Journal of Psychiatry* 120 (1972): 71–78.
5. George L. Engel, "Is Grief a Disease?" *Psychosomatic Medicine* 23 (1961): 18–22.
6. Parkes, *Bereavement*, pp. 197–219.

7. Selby Jacobs and Adrian Ostfeld, "An Epidemiological Review of the Mortality of Bereavement," *Psychosomatic Medicine* 39 (1977): 344–57.

8. R. W. Bartrop et al., "Depressed Lymphocyte Function after Bereavement," *Lancet* 1 (1977): 834–36; and Steven J. Schleifer et al., "Supression of Lymphocyte Stimulation Following Bereavement," *Journal of the American Medical Association* 250 (1983): 374–77.

9. Erwin H. Ackerknecht, *A Short History of Psychiatry*, trans. Sula Wolff, 2d ed., rev. (New York: Hafner Publishing Co., 1968), p. 75.

10. Adolf Meyer, *Psychobiology: A Science of Man* (Springfield, Ill.: Charles C. Thomas, 1957), p. 8.

11. E. E. Southard, "Psychopathology and Neuropathology: The Problems of Teaching and Research Contrasted," *American Journal of Psychology* 23 (1912): 230–35.

12. J. J. C. Smart, "Sensations and Brain Processes," in *The Philosophy of Mind*, ed. V. C. Chappell (Englewood Cliffs, N.J.: Prentice-Hall, 1962), pp. 163–64.

13. C. Lloyd Morgan, *Emergent Evolution* (New York: Henry Holt & Co., 1926), pp. 1–2.

14. Mario Bunge, *The Mind-Body Problem: A Psychobiological Approach* (Oxford: Pergamon Press, 1980), pp. 6–8.

15. Roger Sperry, "Bridging Science and Values: A Unifying View of Mind and Brain," in *Mind and Brain: The Many-Faceted Problems*, ed. Sir John Eccles (Washington: Paragon House, 1982), p. 261.

16. Bunge, *Mind-Body Problem*, p. 217.

17. Karl R. Popper, *Conjectures and Refutations: The Growth of Scientific Knowledge* (London: Routledge & Kegan Paul, 1963), pp. 104–7; and Karl R. Popper and John C. Eccles, *The Self and Its Brain* (Berlin: Springer International, 1977), pp. 171–76.

18. René Descartes, *Descartes: Philosophical Letters*, ed. and trans. Anthony Kenny (Oxford: Clarendon Press, 1970), pp. 69–70.

19. Popper and Eccles, *Self and Brain*.

20. A. M. Turing, "Computing Machinery and Intelligence," in *The Mind's I: Fantasies and Reflections on Self and Soul*, ed. Douglas R. Hofstadter and Daniel C. Dennett (New York: Basic Books, 1981), pp. 53–67.

21. John R. Searle, "Minds, Brains, and Programs," in *The Mind's I*, ed. Hofstadter and Dennett, pp. 369–70.

22. David Bakan, "On the Effect of Mind on Matter," in *Body and Mind: Past, Present, and Future*, ed. R. W. Rieber (New York: Academic Press, 1980), pp. 117–18.

23. Benedict De Spinoza, *On the Improvement of the Understanding, The Ethics, Correspondence*, trans. R. H. M. Elwes (New York: Dover Publications, 1955), p. 86.

24. James W. Papez, "A Proposed Mechanism of Emotion," *Archives of Neurology and Psychiatry* 38 (1937): 725–43.

25. Pierre Flor-Henry, *Cerebral Basis of Psychopathology* (Boston: John Wright-PSG, 1983), p. 45.

26. John Bowlby, "Grief and Mourning in Infancy and Early Childhood," *The Psychoanalytic Study of the Child* 15 (1960): 9–52.

27. Myron A. Hofer, "Studies on How Early Maternal Separation Produces Behavioral Change in Young Rats," *Psychosomatic Medicine* 37 (1975): 245–64.

28. Richard Huntington and Peter Metcalf, *Celebrations of Death* (Cambridge: Cambridge University Press, 1979).

29. Clifford Geertz, *The Religion of Java* (Glencoe, Ill.: Free Press, 1960), p. 73.


Chapter 3. Explanation & Understanding

1. Ann Olivier Bell, ed., *The Diary of Virginia Woolf*, 5 vols. (New York: Harcourt Brace Jovanovich, 1977–84), 1:xv.

2. Leonard Woolf, *Beginning Again: An Autobiography of the Years 1911 to 1918* (New York: Harcourt, Brace & World, 1964), pp. 148–49.

3. Quentin Bell, *Virginia Woolf: A Biography*, 2 vols. (New York: Harcourt Brace Jovanovich, 1972), 2:11.

4. Woolf, *Beginning Again*, pp. 76–77.

5. Nigel Nicolson and Joanne Trautmann, eds., *The Letters of Virginia Woolf*, 6 vols. (New York: Harcourt Brace Jovanovich, 1975–80), 6:481.

6. Bell, *Virginia Woolf*, 1:44.

7. Nicolson and Trautmann, *Letters*, 4:231.

8. Bell, *Virginia Woolf*, 1:90.

9. Paul R. McHugh and Phillip R. Slavney, *The Perspectives of Psychiatry* (Baltimore: Johns Hopkins University Press, 1983), pp. 45–58.

10. Georg Henrik von Wright, *Explanation and Understanding* (Ithaca, N.Y.: Cornell University Press, 1971), pp. 2–3.

11. Max Wartofsky and Richard M. Zaner, "Editorial," *The Journal of Medicine and Science* 5 (1980): 1–7.

12. Karl Jaspers, *General Psychopathology*, trans. J. Hoenig and Marian W. Hamilton (Chicago: The University of Chicago Press, 1963), pp. 27–28.

13. Phillip R. Slavney and Paul R. McHugh, "Life Stories and Meaningful Connections: Reflections on a Clinical Method in Psychiatry and Medicine," *Perspectives in Biology and Medicine* 27 (1984): 279–88.

14. Josef Breuer and Sigmund Freud, "On the Psychical Mechanism of Hysterical Phenomena: Preliminary Communication," in *The Standard Edition of the Complete Psychological Works of Sigmund Freud*, trans. and ed. James Strachey, 24 vols. (London: Hogarth Press and the Institute of Psycho-Analysis, 1953–74), 2:7.

15. Harry Stack Sullivan, *Clinical Studies in Psychiatry*, ed. Helen Swick Perry, Mary Ladd Gawel, and Martha Gibbon (New York: W. W. Norton, 1956), p. 203.

16. Jaspers, *Psychopathology*, pp. 358–59.

17. McHugh and Slavney, *Perspectives*, pp. 53–58.

18. Ibid., pp. 125–40, and Slavney and McHugh, "Life Stories," pp. 279–87.

19. Donald P. Spence, *Narrative Truth and Historical Truth: Meaning and Interpretation in Psychoanalysis* (New York: W. W. Norton, 1982).

20. Nicolson and Trautmann, *Letters*, 6:483.

Chapter 4. Conscious & Unconscious

1. John Locke, *An Essay concerning Human Understanding,* collated and annotated by Alexander Campbell Fraser, 2 vols. (New York: Dover Publications, 1959) 1:138.
2. David Hume, *A Treatise of Human Nature,* ed. L. A. Selby-Bigge (Oxford: Clarendon Press, 1960), pp. 252–53.
3. David Ballin Klein, *The Stream of Consciousness: A Survey* (Lincoln, Neb.: University of Nebraska Press, 1984), p. 11.
4. Jack R. Strange, "A Search for the Sources of the Stream of Consciousness," in *The Stream of Consciousness: Scientific Investigations into the Flow of Human Experience,* ed. Kenneth S. Pope and Jerome L. Singer (New York: Plenum Press, 1978), pp. 11–15.
5. William James, *Essays in Radical Empiricism* (Cambridge: Harvard University Press, 1976), pp. 3–4.
6. John B. Watson, *The Ways of Behaviorism* (New York: Harper & Brothers Publishers, 1928), p. 3.
7. B. F. Skinner, *About Behaviorism* (New York: Alfred A. Knopf, 1974), p. 219.
8. Strange, "Stream of Consciousness," p. 9.
9. Karl Jaspers, *General Psychopathology,* trans. J. Hoenig and Marian B. Hamilton (Chicago: University of Chicago Press, 1963), p. 122.
10. Ralph Barton Perry, "Conceptions and Misconceptions of Consciousness," *The Psychological Review* 11 (1904): 282.
11. Paul R. McHugh and Phillip R. Slavney, *The Perspectives of Psychiatry* (Baltimore: Johns Hopkins University Press, 1983), pp. 30–32.
12. Lancelot Law Whyte, *The Unconscious before Freud* (New York: Basic Books, 1960), pp. 42–43.
13. Locke, *Human Understanding,* 1:129.
14. Whyte, *Unconscious,* p. 64.
15. John Norris, *Cursory Reflections upon a Book Call'd, An Essay concerning Human Understanding,* ed. Gilbert D. McEwen, The Augustan Reprint Society Publication No. 93 (Los Angeles: William Andrews Clark Memorial Library, University of California, 1961), p. 7.
16. G. W. Leibniz, *The Monadology and Other Philosophical Writings,* trans. Robert Latta (Oxford: Clarendon Press, 1898), pp. 370, 376.
17. Richard Hunter and Ida Macalpine, *Three Hundred Years of Psychiatry, 1535–1860: A History Presented in Selected English Texts* (Hartsdale, N.Y.: Carlisle Publishing, 1982), pp. 853–54.
18. Whyte, *Unconscious,* p. 170.
19. Benjamin Libet et al., "Time of Conscious Intention to Act in Relation to Onset of Cerebral Activity (Readiness-Potential): The Unconscious Initiation of a Freely Voluntary Act," *Brain* 106 (1983): 640.
20. Howard Shevrin and Scott Dickman, "The Psychological Unconcious: A Necessary Assumption for All Psychological Theory?," *American Psychologist* 35 (1980): 432.
21. William James, *The Principles of Psychology,* 2 vols. (New York: Henry Holt, 1923), 1:163.
22. Watson, *Behaviorism,* p. 101.
23. Whyte, *Unconscious,* p. 71.

24. Sigmund Freud, "A Note on the Unconscious in Psycho-Analysis," in *The Standard Edition of the Complete Psychological Works of Sigmund Freud,* trans. and ed. James Strachey et al., 24 vols. (London: Hogarth Press and the Institute of Psycho-Analysis, 1953–74), 12:260.

25. Freud, "Fragment of an Analysis of a Case of Hysteria," in *The Standard Edition of the Complete Psychological Works of Sigmund Freud,* trans. and ed. Strachey, 24 vols., 7:114–15.

26. Freud, "Five Lectures on Psycho-Analysis," in *The Standard Edition of the Complete Psychological Works of Sigmund Freud,* trans. and ed. Strachey, 24 vols., 11:37–38.

27. Freud, "New Introductory Lectures on Psycho-Analysis," in *The Standard Edition of the Complete Psychological Works of Sigmund Freud,* trans. and ed. Strachey, 24 vols., 22:70–71.

28. Freud, "Leonardo da Vinci and a Memory of His Childhood," in *The Standard Edition of the Complete Psychological Works of Sigmund Freud,* trans. and ed. Strachey et al., 24 vols., 11:132.

29. Jaspers, *Psychopathology,* p. 10.

30. Freud, "An Outline of Psycho-Analysis," in *The Standard Edition of the Complete Psychological Works of Sigmund Freud,* trans. and ed. Strachey, 24 vols., 23:196.

31. Freud, "New Introductory Lectures," pp. 158–82.

32. Freud, "Outline of Psycho-Analysis," p. 192.

33. Freud, "Project for a Scientific Psychology," in *The Standard Edition of the Complete Psychological Works of Sigmund Freud,* trans. and ed. Strachey, 24 vols., 1:295.

34. Freud, "Outline of Psycho-Analysis," p. 144.

35. Jaspers, *Psychopathology,* p. 244.

36. Freud, "The Question of Lay Analysis: Conversations with an Impartial Person," in *The Standard Edition of the Complete Psychological Works of Sigmund Freud,* trans. and ed. Strachey, 24 vols., 20:248–50.

Chapter 5. Hebraic & Hellenic

1. Karl Jaspers, *General Psychopathology,* trans. J. Hoenig and Marian W. Hamilton (Chicago: University of Chicago Press, 1963), p. 8.

2. Matthew Arnold, *Culture and Anarchy: With Friendship's Garland and Some Literary Essays,* ed. R. H. Super (Ann Arbor: University of Michigan Press, 1960), pp. 167–68.

3. William Barrett, *Irrational Man: A Study in Existential Philosophy* (Garden City, N.Y.: Doubleday Anchor Books, Doubleday, 1962), p. 77.

4. Leon Gibson Hunt, "Growth of Substance Use and Misuse: Some Speculations and Data," in *Control over Intoxicant Use: Pharmacological, Psychological and Social Considerations,* ed. Norman E. Zinberg and Wayne M. Harding (New York: Human Sciences Press, 1982), p. 151.

5. Paul R. McHugh and Phillip R. Slavney, *The Perspectives of Psychiatry* (Baltimore: Johns Hopkins University Press, 1983), pp. 92–97.

6. Jerome D. Frank, *Persuasion and Healing: A Comparative Study of Psychotherapy,* rev. ed. (Baltimore: Johns Hopkins University Press, 1973), p. 314.

7. Leon Salzman, *The Obsessive Personality: Origins, Dynamics and Therapy* (New York: Science House, 1968), pp. 31–32.
8. McHugh and Slavney, *Perspectives,* pp. 89–90.
9. Ibid., pp. 125–40.
10. Donald P. Spence, *Narrative Truth and Historical Truth: Meaning and Interpretation in Psychoanalysis* (New York: W. W. Norton, 1982), p. 293.
11. Phillip R. Slavney and Paul R. McHugh, "The Life-Story Method in Psychotherapy and Psychiatric Education: The Development of Confidence," *American Journal of Psychotherapy* 39 (1985): 57–67.
12. Hilde Bruch, *Learning Psychotherapy* (Cambridge: Harvard University Press, 1974), p. 85.
13. Frank, *Persuasion,* p. 325.
14. E. H. Uhlenhuth and David B. Duncan, "Subjective Change with Medical Student Therapists: I. Course of Relief in Psychoneurotic Outpatients," *Archives of General Psychiatry* 18 (1968): 428–38.
15. Frank, *Persuasion,* p. 325.

## Chapter 6. Patient & Client

1. Holly Skodol Wilson and Carol Rem Kneisl, *Psychiatric Nursing,* 2d ed. (Menlo Park, Calif.: Addison-Wesley Publishing Co., Nursing Division, 1983), p. 870.
2. Wilbert E. Moore, in collaboration with Gerald E. Rosenblum, *The Professions: Rules and Roles* (New York: Russell Sage Foundation, 1970), p. 5.
3. William F. May, "Code and Covenant or Philanthropy and Contract," in *Ethics in Medicine: Historical Perspectives and Contemporary Concerns,* ed. Stanley Joel Reiser, Arthur J. Dyck, and William J. Curran (Cambridge: MIT Press, 1977), pp. 71–72.
4. James E. Giles, *Medical Ethics: A Patient-Centered Approach* (Cambridge, Mass.: Schenkman Publishing Co., 1983), p. 218.
5. May, "Code and Covenant," p. 72.
6. Edmund D. Pellegrino, "Toward a Reconstruction of Medical Morality: The Primacy of the Act of Profession and the Fact of Illness," *Journal of Medicine and Philosophy* 4 (1979): 32–56.
7. Edmund D. Pellegrino, "The Physician-Patient Relationship in Preventive Medicine: Reply to Robert Dickman," *Journal of Medicine and Philosophy* 5 (1980): 208–12.
8. Pellegrino, "Reconstruction of Medical Morality," p. 44.

## Chapter 7. Autonomy & Paternalism

1. Leonard Woolf, *Beginning Again: An Autobiography of the Years 1911 to 1918* (New York: Harcourt, Brace & World, 1964), pp. 156–57.
2. Dennis J. Horan and David Mall, eds., *Death, Dying, and Euthanasia* (Washington, D.C.: University Publications of America, 1977); Ernan McMullan, ed., *Death and Decision* (Boulder, Colo.: Westview Press, 1978); Marc D. Basson, ed., *Rights and Responsibilities in Modern Medicine: The Second Volume in a Series on Ethics, Humanism, and*

*Medicine* (New York: Alan R. Liss, 1981); and Benedict M. Ashley and Kevin D. O'Rourke, *Health Care Ethics: A Theological Analysis,* 2d ed., (St. Louis: Catholic Health Association of the United States, 1982).

3. Joseph Fletcher, *Humanhood: Essays in Biomedical Ethics* (Buffalo, N.Y.: Prometheus Books, 1979), p. 175.

4. Thomas Szasz, *The Theology of Medicine: The Political-Philosophical Foundations of Medical Ethics* (Baton Rouge: Louisiana State University Press, 1977), p. 84.

5. Bruce L. Miller, "Autonomy & the Refusal of Lifesaving Treatment," *The Hastings Center Report* 11 (1981): 24.

6. John Kleinig, *Paternalism* (Totowa, N.J.: Rowman and Allanheld, 1984), p. 13.

7. John Stuart Mill, *The Philosophy of John Stuart Mill: Ethical, Political and Religious,* ed. Marshall Cohen (New York: Modern Library, 1961), pp. 196–97.

8. Thomas S. Szasz and Marc H. Hollender, "A Contribution to the Philosophy of Medicine: The Basic Models of the Doctor-Patient Relationship," *A.M.A. Archives of Internal Medicine* 97 (1956): 585–92.

9. Eric J. Cassell, "What Is the Function of Medicine?," in *Death and Decision,* ed. Ernan McMullan (Boulder, Colo.: Westview Press, 1978), pp. 35–44.

10. Gerald Dworkin, "Paternalism," in *Morality and the Law,* ed. Richard A. Wasserstrom (Belmont, Calif.: Wadsworth Publishing Co., 1971), pp. 107–26; Miller, "Autonomy," pp.22–28; and Ruth Macklin, "Treatment Refusals: Autonomy, Paternalism, and the 'Best Interest' of the Patient," in *Ethical Questions in Brain and Behavior: Problems and Opportunities,* ed. Donald W. Pfaff (New York: Springer-Verlag, 1983), pp. 41–56.

11. Cassell, "Function of Medicine," pp. 40–41.

12. Mark S. Komrad, "A Defence of Medical Paternalism: Maximising Patients' Autonomy," *Journal of Medical Ethics* 9 (1983): 38–44.

13. Cassell, "Function of Medicine," p. 40.

14. Paul R. McHugh and Phillip R. Slavney, *The Perspectives of Psychiatry* (Baltimore: Johns Hopkins University Press, 1983), p. 102.

15. Brian Barraclough et al., "A Hundred Cases of Suicide: Clinical Aspects," *British Journal of Psychiatry* 125 (1974): 355–73.

16. Eli Robins, *The Final Months: A Study of the Lives of 134 Persons Who Committed Suicide* (New York: Oxford University Press, 1981).

17. Barraclough et al., "Hundred Cases of Suicide," p. 371.

18. Cassell, "Function of Medicine," p. 40.

19. Woolf, *Beginning Again,* pp. 162–64.

20. Nigel Nicolson and Joanne Trautmann, eds., *The Letters of Virginia Woolf,* 6 vols. (New York: Harcourt Brace Jovanovich, 1975–80), 1:143.

Chapter 8. The Ambiguity of Psychiatry: A Methodological Resolution

1. Karl Jaspers, *General Psychopathology,* trans. J. Hoenig and Marian W. Hamilton (Chicago: University of Chicago Press, 1963), pp. 765–66.

2. George L. Engel, "The Need for a New Medical Model: A Challenge for Biomedicine," *Science* 196 (1977): 129–36; and "The Clinical Application

of the Biopsychosocial Model," *American Journal of Psychiatry* 137 (1980): 535–44.

3. Paul R. McHugh and Phillip R. Slavney, *The Perspectives of Psychiatry* (Baltimore: Johns Hopkins University Press, 1983).

4. Antonio Lobo, *Prólogo a la edición castellana,* in Paul R. McHugh and Phillip R. Slavney, *Perspectivas de la Psiquiatría,* trans. Antonio Lobo (Barcelona: Masson, 185), p. xi.

# Index